Color Atlas of
Small Animal Anatomy:
The Essentials

T0340716

Color Atlas of
Small Animal Anatomy:
The Essentials

Thomas O. McCracken, MS, PhD (Hon)
Professor Anatomy
University of Medicine and Health Sciences/
International University of Nursing
Basseterre, St. Kitts
West Indies

Robert A. Kainer, DVM, MS
Professor Emeritus of Anatomy
College of Veterinary Medicine and Biomedical Sciences
Colorado State University
Fort Collins, Colorado

David Carlson, Illustrator
President/Creative Director
BioGraphix, LLC
Windsor, Colorado

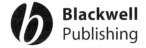
Blackwell
Publishing

Blackwell Publishing Professional
2121 State Avenue, Ames, Iowa 50014, USA

Orders:	**1-800-862-6657**
Office:	**1-515-292-0140**
Fax:	**1-515-292-3348**
Web site:	**www.blackwellprofessional.com**

Blackwell Publishing Ltd
9600 Garsington Road, Oxford OX4 2DQ, UK
Tel.: +44 (0)1865 776868

Blackwell Publishing Asia
550 Swanston Street, Carlton, Victoria 3053, Australia
Tel.: +61 (0)3 8359 1011

Authorization to photocopy items for internal or personal use, or the internal or personal use of specific clients, is granted by Blackwell Publishing, provided that the base fee is paid directly to the Copyright Clearance Center, 222 Rosewood Drive, Danvers, MA 01923. For those organizations that have been granted a photocopy license by CCC, a separate system of payments has been arranged. The fee codes for users of the Transactional Reporting Service are ISBN-13: 978-0-8138-1608-1/2008.

First edition, 2008

Library of Congress Cataloging-in-Publication Data

McCracken, Thomas.
    Color atlas of small animal anatomy : the essentials / Thomas O. McCracken, Robert A. Kainer.
        p. ; cm.
    Includes index.
    ISBN-13: 978-0-8138-1608-1 (alk. paper)
    ISBN-10: 0-8138-1608-4 (alk. paper)
    1. Veterinary anatomy—Atlases. 2. Cats—Anatomy—Atlases. 3. Dogs—Anatomy—Atlases. I. Kainer, Robert A. II. Title.
    [DNLM: 1. Anatomy, Veterinary—Atlases. 2. Cats—anatomy & histology—Atlases. 3. Dogs—anatomy & histology—Atlases. 4. Guinea Pigs—anatomy & histology—Atlases. 5. Rabbits—anatomy & histology—Atlases. 6. Rats—anatomy & histology—Atlases. SF 761 M478c 2008]
    SF751.M33 2008
    636.089'1—dc22
                                                                2007029634

SKY10073208_041724

The last digit is the print number:

ACKNOWLEDGMENTS

The authors express their gratitude to Dennis Madden, diener at Colorado State University College of Veterinary Medicine, for assistance with specimens for dissection. Special thanks to David Carlson on his accurate and artistic interpretation of the original black & white line drawings into beautiful color plates.

The patience and counsel of the staff at Blackwell Publishing is gratefully acknowledged.

Several illustrations were redrawn from the following sources:

Evans, H.E. (ed.): Miller's Anatomy of the Dog, 3rd ed., Philadelphia, W.B. Saunders, l993. Figure 9-7

Hudson, L.C., Hamilton W.P.: Atlas of Feline Anatomy for Veterinarians, W.B. Saunders, 1993

The following publications were used for general reference:

Boyd, J.S.: A Color Atlas of Clinical Anatomy of the Dog and Cat, London, Mosby-Wolfe, 1991

Budras, K-D, Fricke, W., McCarthy, P.H.: Anatomy of the Dog—An Illustrated Text, 3rd Ed., London, Mosby-Wolfe, 1994

Chiasson, R.B.: Laboratory Anatomy of the White Rat, Boston, McGraw-Hill, 1994

Cooper, G., Schiller, A. L.: Anatomy of the Guinea Pig, Boston, Harvard University Press, 1975

Done, S.H., Evans, S.A., Strickland, N.C.: Color Atlas of Veterinary Anatomy, Vol. 3, The Dog and Cat, London, Mosby-Wolfe, 1996

Ellenberger, W., Dittrich, H., Baum, H., Brown L.S. (ed.): An Atlas of Animal Anatomy for Artists, New York, Dover Publications, 1956

Evans, H.E., (ed.): Miller's Anatomy of the Dog, 3rd Ed., Philadelphia, W.B. Saunders, 1993

Hudson, L.C., Hamilton W.P.: Atlas of Feline Anatomy for Veterinarians, W.B. Saunders, 1993

McLaughlin C., Chiasson, R. B.: Laboratory Anatomy of the Rabbit, Boston, McGraw-Hill, 1992

Popesko, P.: A Color Atlas of The Anatomy of Small Laboratory Animals volume 1 (Rabbit, Guinea Pig) & volume 2 (Rat, Mouse, Hamster) Wolfe, 1992

Popesko, P.: Atlas of Topographical Anatomy of the Domestic Animals, Philadelphia, W. B. Saunders, 1979

Walker, F.W. Jr., Homberger, D.G.: Anatomy & Dissection of the Rat, New York, W.H. Freeman and Company, 1997

Wells, T.A.G., The Rat, Dover Publications, Inc., 1964

CONTENTS

SECTION 1   THE DOG

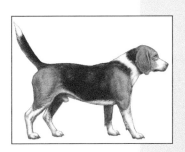

SECTION 2   THE CAT

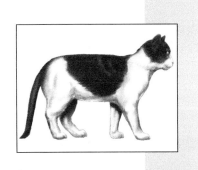

SECTION 3   THE RABBIT

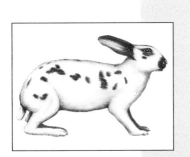

SECTION 4   THE RAT

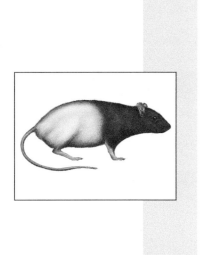
SECTION 5   THE GUINEA PIG

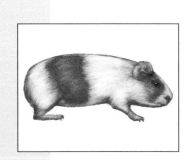

INTRODUCTION

The Color Atlas of Small Animal Anatomy: *The Essentials* is not a complete, detailed anatomic atlas. Instead it presents topographic relationships of the major organs of the dog, cat, rabbit, rat, and guinea pig in a simple yet technically accurate format. Throughout most of the *Atlas*, a male and a female of a given species are on facing pages. The majority of the plates contain information on the entire body. Some plates are confined to a region; a few contain organs isolated from the rest of the body. Whereas most systems (e.g., digestive and reproductive) are presented for each animal, other systems are included only for some species to illustrate general anatomic patterns. Structures common to the various animals are labeled several times; other structures are labeled on only one or two species, usually emphasizing specific anatomy (the anatomy peculiar to a certain species).

Small animal specialists and researchers have advised the authors on special plates for individual animals.

The *Atlas* is intended for use by individuals at different stages of their education, serving as a survey of the specific anatomy of the different small animals. Advanced 4-H club members, high school vocational agriculture students, and college students studying veterinary medical technology, veterinary medicine, animal science, and wildlife biology can use this *Atlas* as an introduction to the anatomy of common small / laboratory animals. The *Atlas* can also serve as a reference for dog and cat breeders and trainers, as well as laboratory technicians and researchers. It will provide a quick review for persons with previous training in anatomy and will be an invaluable aid for the professional—e. g., a veterinarian or animal scientist—in explaining to a client some aspect of anatomy that pertains to an animal's condition and needs.

The following introductory pages provide the reader with a background in nomenclature and anatomic orientation.

ANIMAL CLASSIFICATION

Dog (*Canis lupus familiaris*). The dog (*Order Carnivora*) is a domesticated wolf in the family Canidae, to which the jackal and fox also belong. Two characteristics distinguish the dog from other canids and, indeed, from all other animal species. The first is its worldwide distribution in close association with humans. The second is the enormous amount of variability found within the subspecies.

The anatomy of dogs varies tremendously from breed to breed. Some basic physical characteristics are identical among all dogs, from the smallest to the largest; most but not all dogs have long muzzles, large canine teeth, and long tails. Like most predatory mammals, the dog has powerful muscles, a cardiovascular system that supports both sprinting and endurance, and teeth for catching, holding, and tearing. Dogs have disconnected shoulder bones (no collar bone) that allow a greater stride length for running and leaping. They walk on four toes, front and back, and have vestigial dewclaws (dog thumbs) on their forelimbs and hind limbs. Dogs exhibit a diverse array of fur coats; they range from different coat textures, colors, markings, and patterns.

Cat (*Felis catus*). Cat is the name applied broadly to the mammals in the order Carnivora, family Felidae, and specifically to the domestic cat. All cats have rounded heads, short muzzles, large eyes, sensitive tactile hairs around the mouth, and erect pointed ears. They have short, wide jaws equipped with long canine teeth and strong cheek teeth with sharp cutting edges. Their tongues are coated with sharp backward-facing papillae that aid in drinking and grooming. The ends of the toes bear strong, sharp, curved claws. The claws are completely retractile, being withdrawn into protective cutaneous sheaths when not in use, a distinguishing feature of the cat family. Cats have long tails which they use for balance. The musculo-skeletal system is extremely flexible, allowing cats to arch and twist their bodies in a variety of ways. Most cats have good vision and are able to see well in very dim light; their color vision is weak. Their sense of hearing is excellent; their sense of smell is not as acute as that in dogs. Cats may be solid-colored or have patches or shadings of a second color; some common patterns are: tabby, tortoiseshell, and calico, among others.

Rabbit. The European rabbit (*Oryctolagus cuniculus*) is in the order Lagomorpha which also includes the hare and the pika. These animals have two large upper first incisor teeth with two small second incisors behind them. This immediately distinguishes lagomorphs from rodents. Other distinguishing features are short tails and large hind limbs and feet adapted for running or jumping. In most, the length of the ears is considerably greater than the width.The rabbit skeleton is light, making up only 7-8% of body weight. The forelimbs are short and fine, in contrast to the long and powerful hind limbs. The plantar surface of the hind limb from the tarsus distad is in contact with the ground at rest. The spine is naturally curved.

The upper lip of the rabbit is cleft (hare lip). Rabbits have a total of 6 incisors (the teeth you see in the front), two sets upper and one set lower, and no canine teeth. The cheek teeth consist of three upper premolars and three upper molars, and two lower premolars and two lower molars on each side.

Although usage varies, the term rabbit generally refers to small, running animals which give birth to altricial (naked and blind) young, while hare refers to larger, hopping forms, with longer ears and limbs whose young are precocious (born furred and open-eyed). They have acute senses of smell and hearing.

Rat. Rats are rodents with stout bodies, usually having a pointed muzzle, a long, slender, naked tail, and dexterous forepaws. Rat refers particularly to the two species of house rat—the brown, or *Norway*, rat (*Rattus norwegicus*) and *Rattus rattus*, the *black*, *roof*, or *Alexandrine*, rat. Besides the house rats, the genus *Rattus* contains several hundred wild-living species.

The brown rat is the larger of the two, growing up to 10 in. (25 cm) long excluding the naked, scaly tail, and sometimes weighing more than a pound (.5 kg). It is commonly brown with whitish underparts and pink ears, feet, and tail. The laboratory white rat is an albino strain of the brown rat. The black rat is commonly dark gray. It reaches a maximum length of 8 in. (20 cm) and has a longer tail and larger ears than the brown rat. As with the rabbit, the rat's teeth grow continually during its life.

Guinea pig. The guinea pig (*cavy*, *Cavia porcellus*). It is a South American rodent unrelated to the pig; the name may refer to its shrill squeal. The guinea pig is a small, burrowing rodent that has a compact body. They have rounded bodies, large heads, and blunt noses and reach a length of 6 to

10 in. (15-25 cm) and a weight of 1 to 2 lb (450-900 grams). The guinea pig's rapid reproductive rate and high resistance to disease make it a valuable laboratory animal. It has small ears and eyes, a small snout with sensory tactile hairs on each side, and no tail. Like most rodents, it has two upper and lower teeth at the front of the mouth which continue to grow throughout its life. It has short limbs and small feet with claws; the forefeet have four toes/claws, but the hind feet have only three.

There are a number of varieties of guinea pig; their coats can have short or long smooth hair with a great variety of color combinations, mainly mixtures of black and white and many shades of brown.

GENERAL TERMINOLOGY

With some exceptions, particularly for some muscles wherein traditional Latin names are used, the terminology in this *Atlas* conforms to English translations of Latin terms in the *Nomina Anatomica Veterinaria (N.A.V.)*, 3rd ed., 1983. In compliance with the intent of *N.A.V.*, nomenclature will be consistent for all species. Common terms and laboratory terms are used in some plates. Abbreviations for organs in this *Atlas* include: a, artery; b, bone; j, joint; lig., ligament; ln., lymph node; m, muscle; n, nerve; v, vein. Double letters indicate the plural form of these words (e. g., aa, arteries). Positional and directional terms, body planes, and the extent of body cavities are used to indicate the location of parts of the body and functional change in position.

POSITIONAL AND DIRECTIONAL TERMS

The following terms are illustrated on the accompanying illustration of the dog. **Dorsal** and **ventral** are opposite terms indicating relative locations toward the back (L., dorsum) or belly (L., venter). Above the knee (carpus) and the hock (tarsus) and from the belly to the back, a structure located closer to the cranium (skull case) is **cranial** to another structure, and a structure located toward the tail (L., cauda) is **caudal** to another. On the head, the term **rostral** indicates a structure closer to the nose (L., rostrum).

 Proximal indicates a location toward the attached end of a limb; **distal** indicates a location toward the free end of a limb, that is, further from the trunk. Distal to and including the carpus, **dorsal** replaces cranial; **palmar** replaces caudal. Distal to and including the hock, dorsal replaces cranial, and **plantar** replaces caudal.

 Positional adverbs end in -al; directional adverbs, in -ad. For example, one structure is proximal to another; a tendon extends distad to join another. A vein courses proximad.

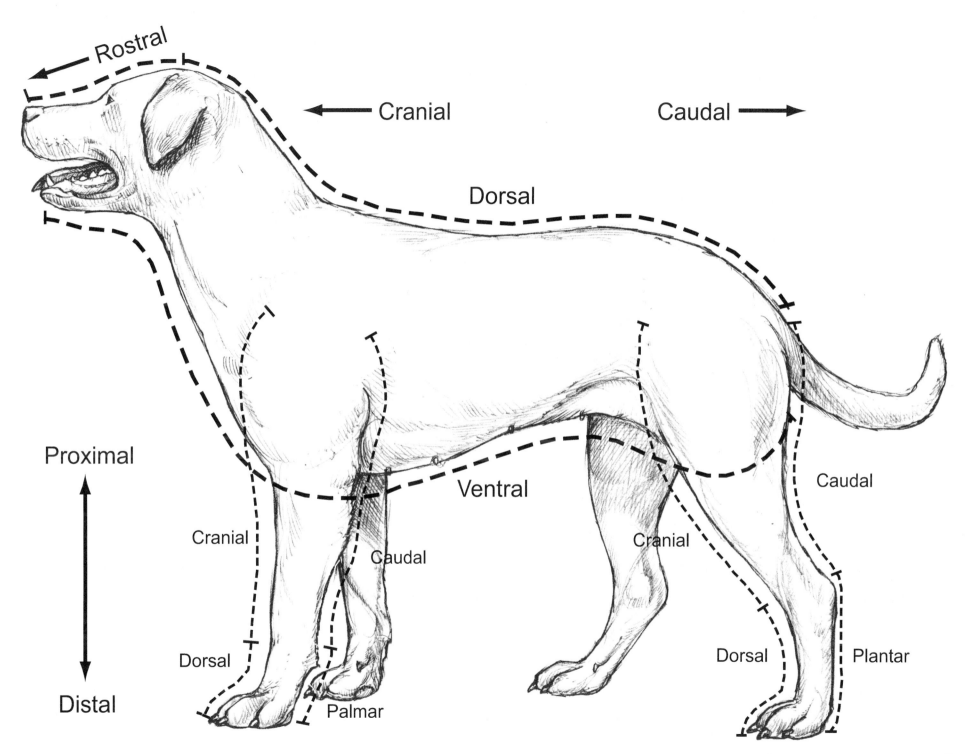

Rostral

Cranial

Caudal

Dorsal

Proximal

Ventral

Caudal

Cranial

Cranial

Distal

Dorsal

Caudal

Dorsal

Plantar

Palmar

BODY PLANES

Illustrations of the dog are used to illustrate body planes. The **median plane** (L., medius, middle) divides the animal body into right and left halves. A **sagittal plane** (L., sagitta, arrow) is any plane parallel to the median plane. **Medial** and **lateral** (L., latus, side) are positional terms relative to the median plane. Medial structures are located closer to the median plane. Lateral structures lie away from the median plane, that is, toward the side. They extend laterad (directional term). A **transverse plane** passes through the head, trunk, or limb perpendicular to the part's long axis. A **dorsal plane** (also called a **frontal plane**) is a longitudinal plane that passes through the body parallel to its dorsal surface at right angles to the median plane.

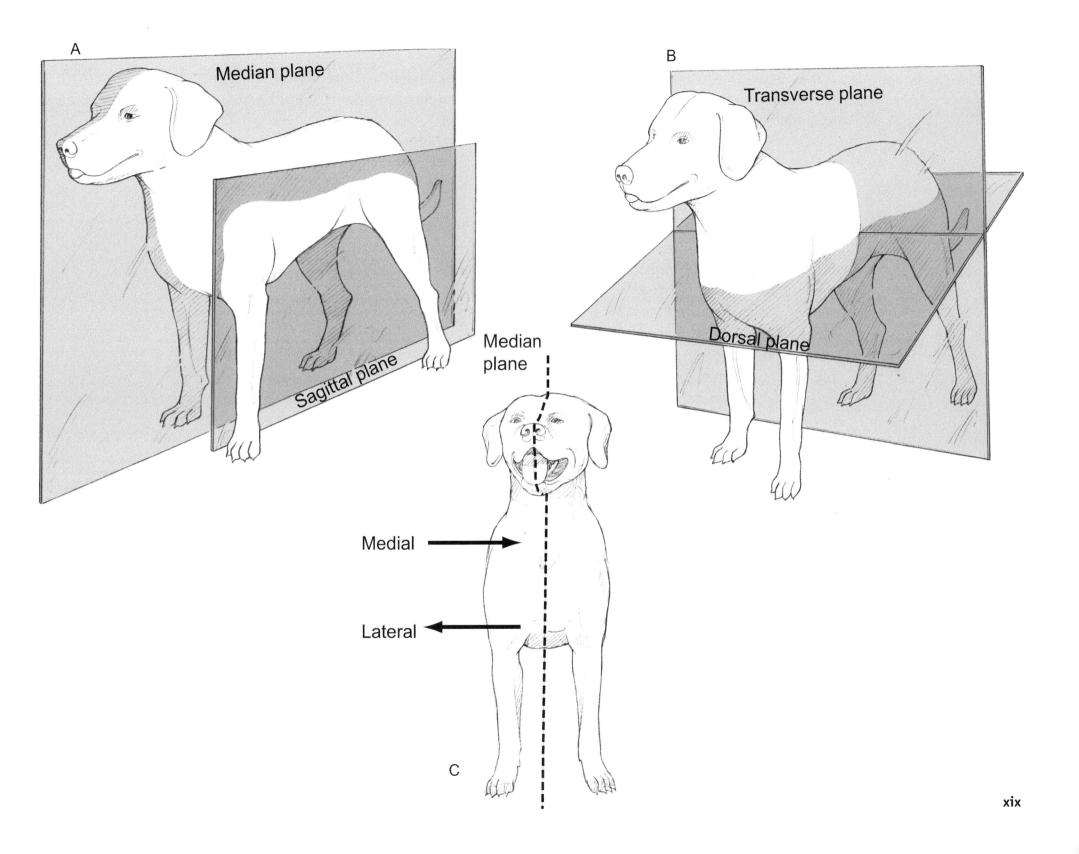

A

Median plane

Sagittal plane

B

Transverse plane

Dorsal plane

Median plane

Medial

Lateral

C

BODY CAVITIES AND MEMBRANES

A diagrammatic illustration of the female dog illustrates the **thoracic, abdominal,** and **pelvic cavities** and the serous membranes—**peritoneum, pleura,** and **pericardium**—that line body cavities and suspend organs.

The peritoneum consists of three continuous parts. The **parietal peritoneum** (L., paries, wall) lines the abdominal cavity and the cranial part of the pelvic cavity. **Connecting peritoneum** reflects from the parietal peritoneum and suspends organs in a double fold containing vessels and nerves as it extends to an organ. The connecting peritoneum is indicated by mes- (G., mesos, middle) plus the Latin or Greek name of the organ. An example is **mesentery**: mes- plus enteron (G. intestine). Peritoneal ligaments suspend and support—e.g., falciform ligament of the liver. **Visceral peritoneum** is continuous with connecting peritoneum, encircling a viscus (Latin for a large, internal organ; plural, **viscera**).

The musculomembranous **diaphragm** is covered with parietal peritoneum on its abdominal surface and parietal (diaphragmatic) pleura on its thoracic surface.

The **pleurae** are two continuous serous membranes, each forming a pleural sac. The **parietal pleura** line each half of the thoracic cavity. **Mediastinal pleura** is connecting pleura on each side enclosing the **mediastium**, a space containing the heart, esophagus, trachea, blood vessels, lymph nodes and ducts, thymus, nerves, and adipose tissue. **Visceral (pulmonary) pleura** covers each lung.

The **pericardium** is the heart sac. **Visceral** pericardium (also called epicardium) covers the heart and reflects around the base of the heart and great vessels to become continuous with the **parietal pericardium.** The latter is attached to a fibrous layer, the fibrous pericardium.

The serous cavities—**peritoneal cavity, pleural cavity,** and **pericardial cavity**—are potential spaces between parietal and visceral membranes containing lubricating serous fluids named for each cavity or sac.

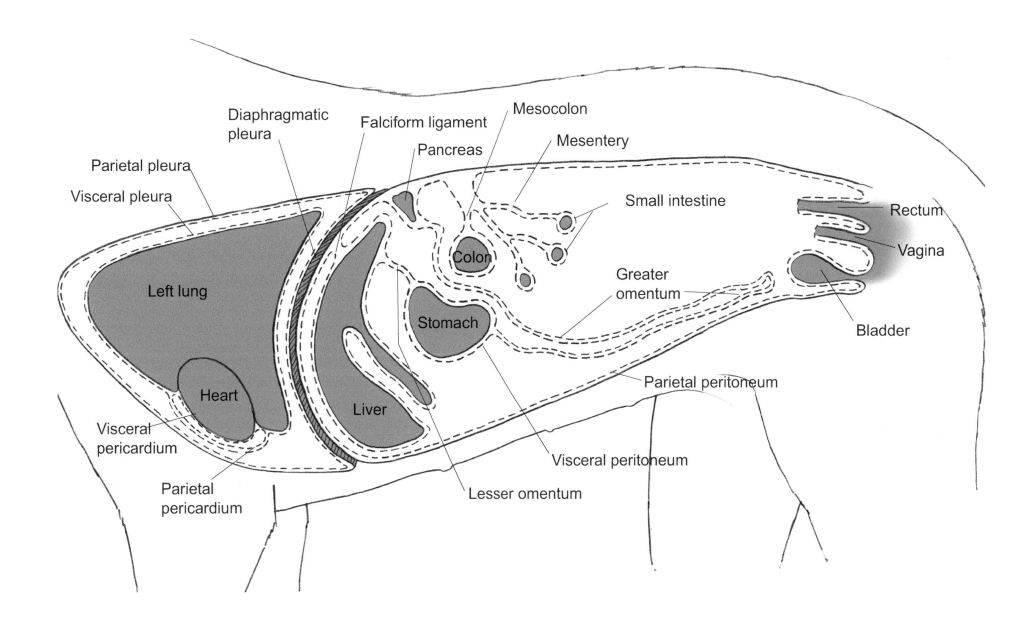

Diaphragmatic pleura

Falciform ligament

Mesocolon

Pancreas

Mesentery

Parietal pleura

Visceral pleura

Small intestine

Rectum

Colon

Vagina

Greater omentum

Left lung

Stomach

Bladder

Heart

Liver

Parietal peritoneum

Visceral pericardium

Visceral peritoneum

Parietal pericardium

Lesser omentum

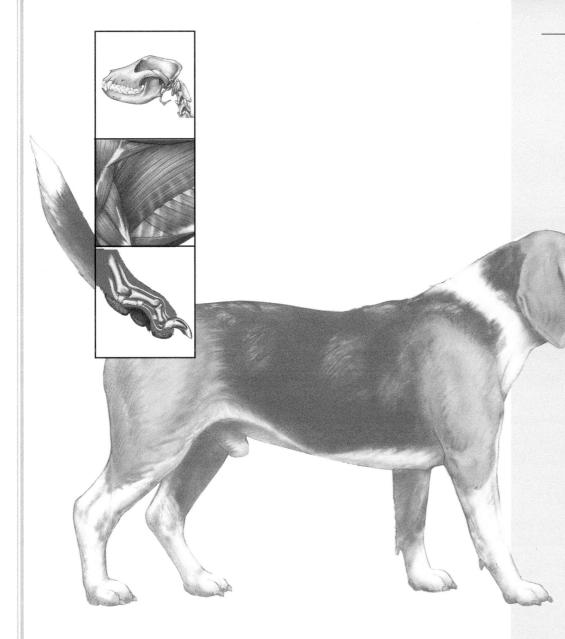

SECTION 1　THE DOG

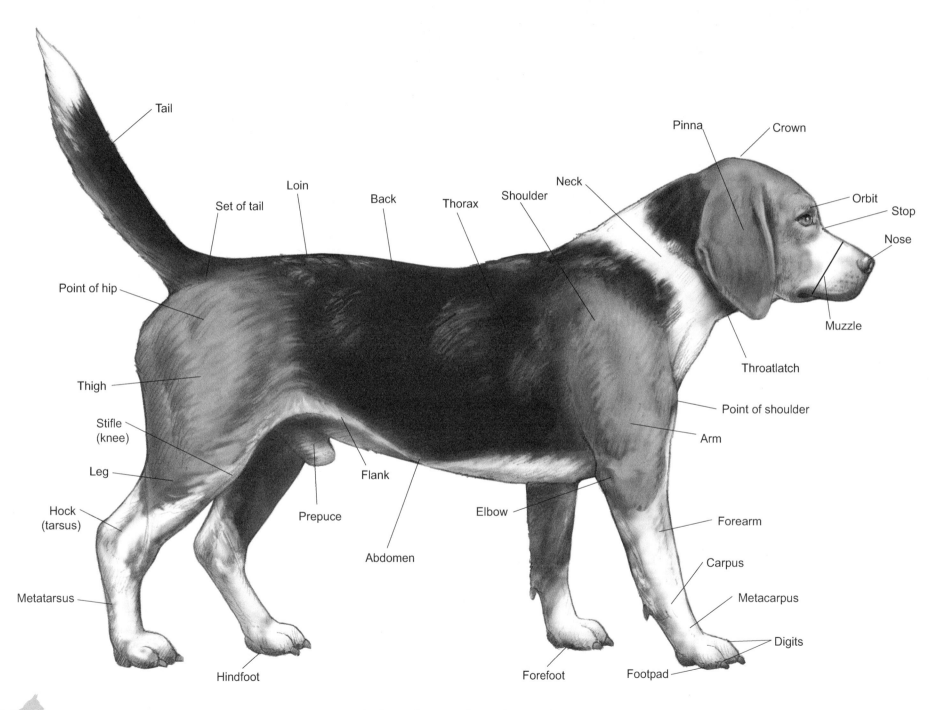

PLATE 1.1   Right lateral view of a male Beagle dog.

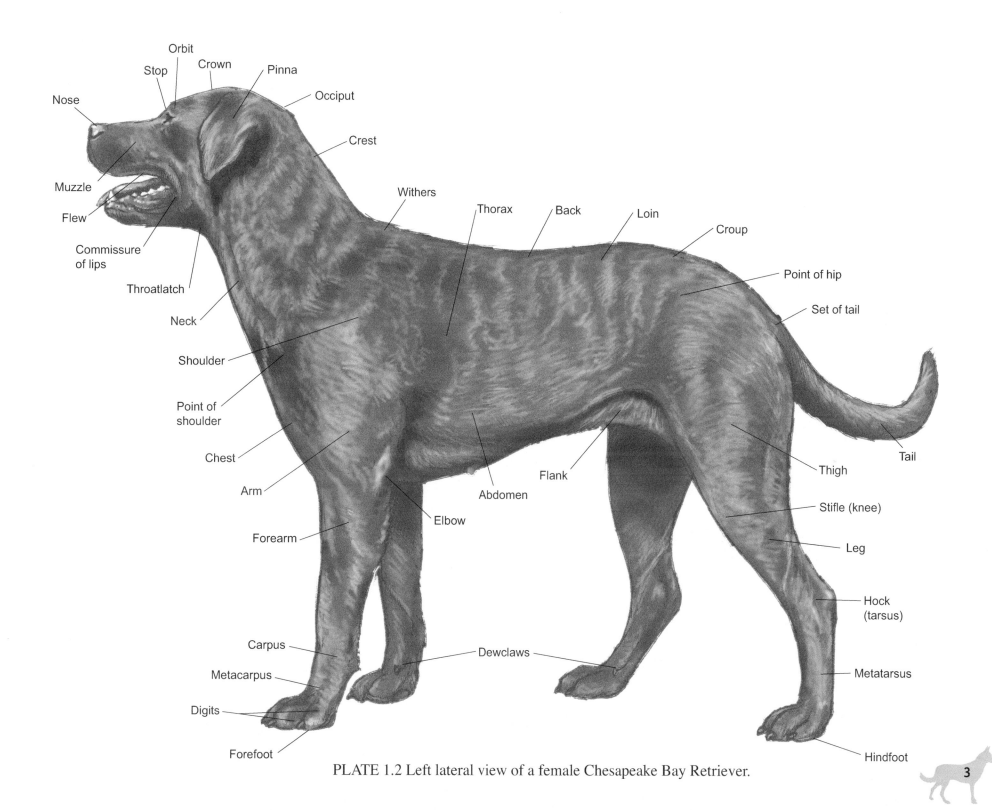

PLATE 1.2 Left lateral view of a female Chesapeake Bay Retriever.

3

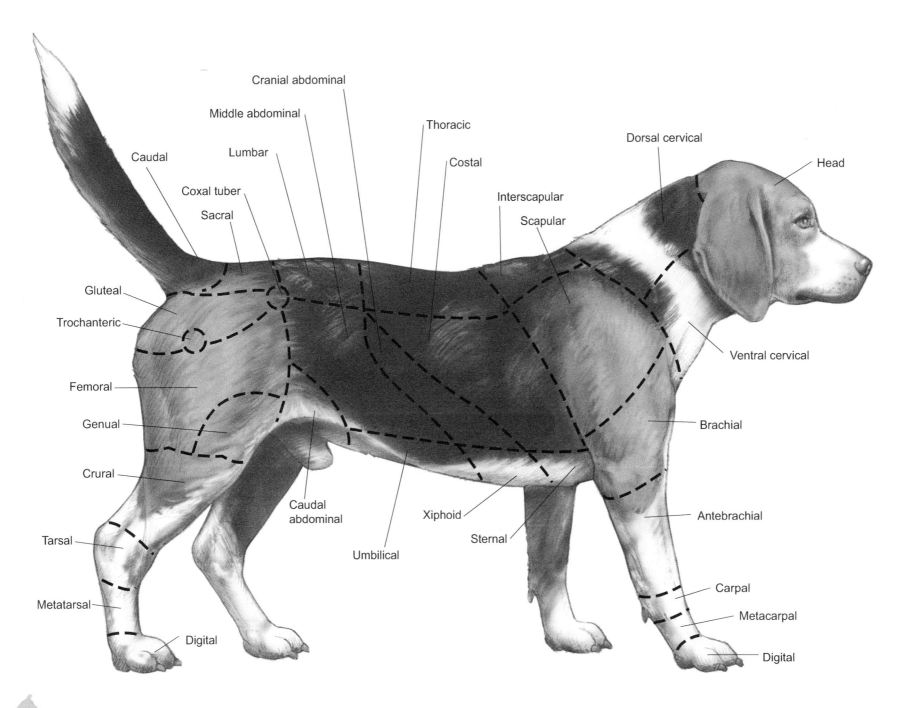

Cranial abdominal

Middle abdominal

Lumbar

Caudal

Coxal tuber

Sacral

Thoracic

Costal

Dorsal cervical

Head

Interscapular

Scapular

Gluteal

Trochanteric

Femoral

Genual

Ventral cervical

Crural

Brachial

Caudal abdominal

Xiphoid

Umbilical

Sternal

Antebrachial

Tarsal

Metatarsal

Carpal

Metacarpal

Digital

Digital

PLATE 1.3 Body regions.

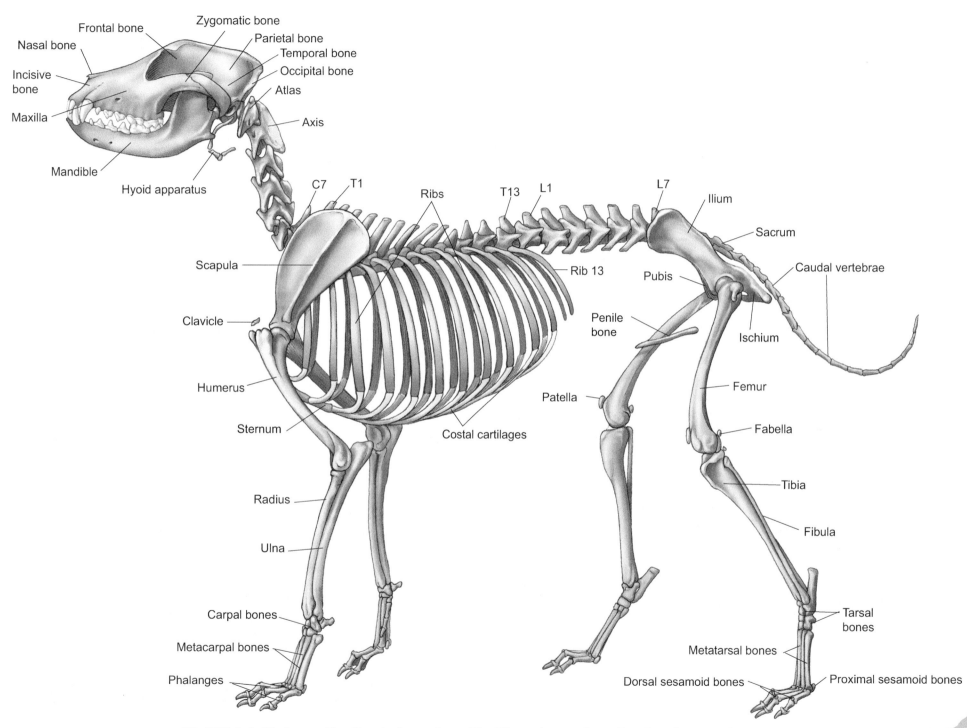

Frontal bone
Zygomatic bone
Nasal bone
Parietal bone
Incisive bone
Temporal bone
Occipital bone
Maxilla
Atlas
Mandible
Axis
Hyoid apparatus
C7
T1
Ribs
T13
L1
L7
Ilium
Scapula
Sacrum
Rib 13
Caudal vertebrae
Clavicle
Pubis
Penile bone
Ischium
Humerus
Femur
Patella
Sternum
Fabella
Costal cartilages
Radius
Tibia
Fibula
Ulna
Carpal bones
Tarsal bones
Metacarpal bones
Metatarsal bones
Phalanges
Dorsal sesamoid bones
Proximal sesamoid bones

PLATE 1.4 Skeleton; C = Cervical vertebrae, T = Thoracic vertebrae, L = Lumbar vertebrae.

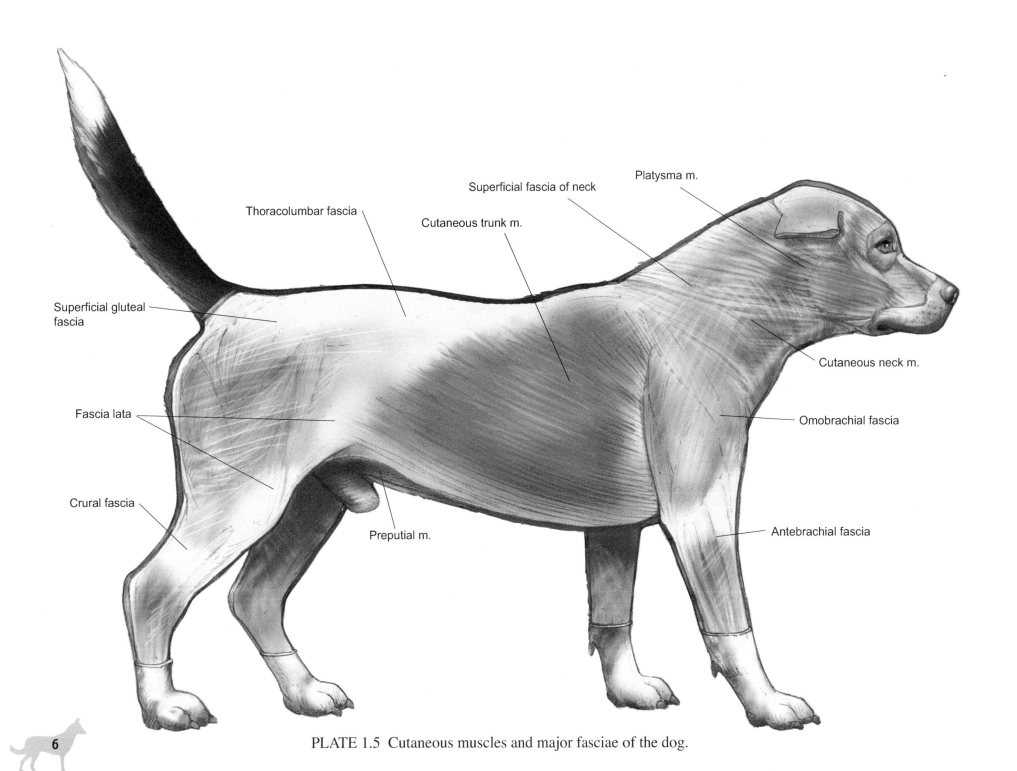

Thoracolumbar fascia

Superficial fascia of neck

Platysma m.

Cutaneous trunk m.

Superficial gluteal fascia

Cutaneous neck m.

Fascia lata

Omobrachial fascia

Crural fascia

Preputial m.

Antebrachial fascia

PLATE 1.5 Cutaneous muscles and major fasciae of the dog.

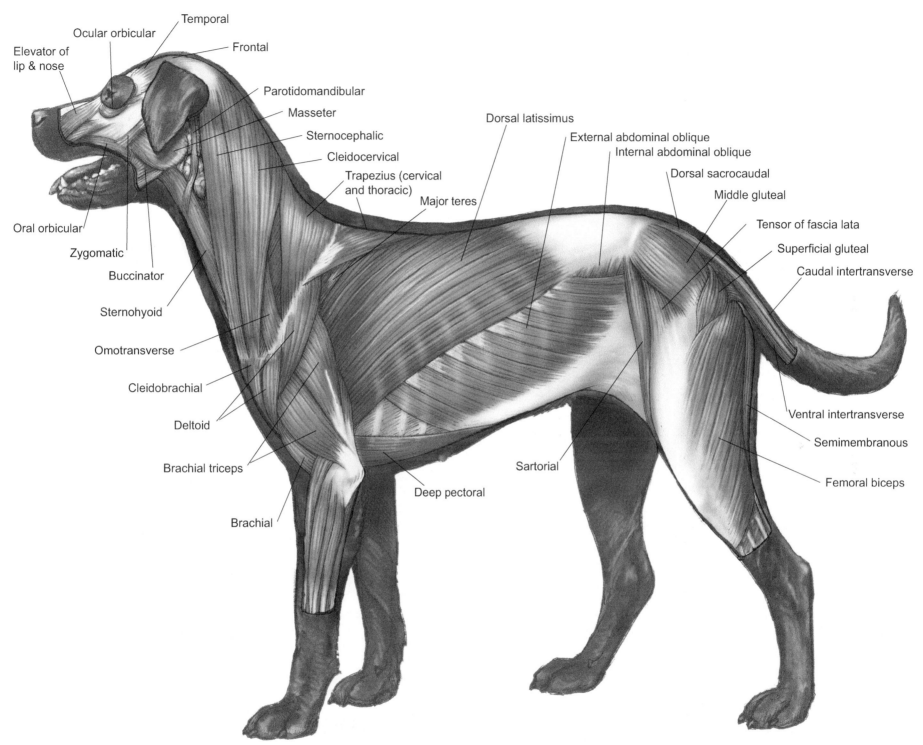

Elevator of lip & nose

Ocular orbicular

Temporal

Frontal

Parotidomandibular

Masseter

Sternocephalic

Cleidocervical

Trapezius (cervical and thoracic)

Major teres

Dorsal latissimus

External abdominal oblique

Internal abdominal oblique

Dorsal sacrocaudal

Middle gluteal

Tensor of fascia lata

Superficial gluteal

Caudal intertransverse

Oral orbicular

Zygomatic

Buccinator

Sternohyoid

Omotransverse

Cleidobrachial

Deltoid

Brachial triceps

Brachial

Deep pectoral

Sartorial

Ventral intertransverse

Semimembranous

Femoral biceps

PLATE 1.6 Superficial muscles of the bitch.

7

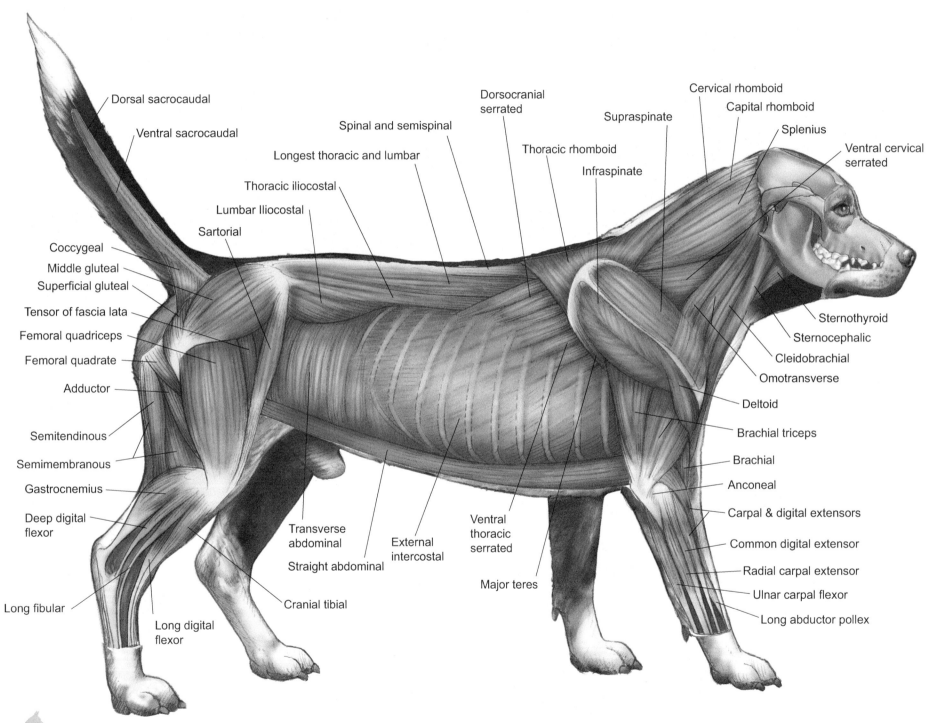

Dorsal sacrocaudal

Ventral sacrocaudal

Spinal and semispinal

Dorsocranial serrated

Longest thoracic and lumbar

Thoracic rhomboid

Cervical rhomboid

Capital rhomboid

Splenius

Supraspinate

Ventral cervical serrated

Thoracic iliocostal

Infraspinate

Lumbar Iliocostal

Coccygeal

Sartorial

Middle gluteal

Superficial gluteal

Tensor of fascia lata

Femoral quadriceps

Femoral quadrate

Sternothyroid

Sternocephalic

Cleidobrachial

Adductor

Omotransverse

Deltoid

Semitendinous

Brachial triceps

Semimembranous

Brachial

Gastrocnemius

Anconeal

Carpal & digital extensors

Deep digital flexor

Transverse abdominal

Ventral thoracic serrated

Common digital extensor

Straight abdominal

External intercostal

Radial carpal extensor

Long fibular

Major teres

Ulnar carpal flexor

Long digital flexor

Cranial tibial

Long abductor pollex

8

PLATE 1.7 Deep muscles of the dog.

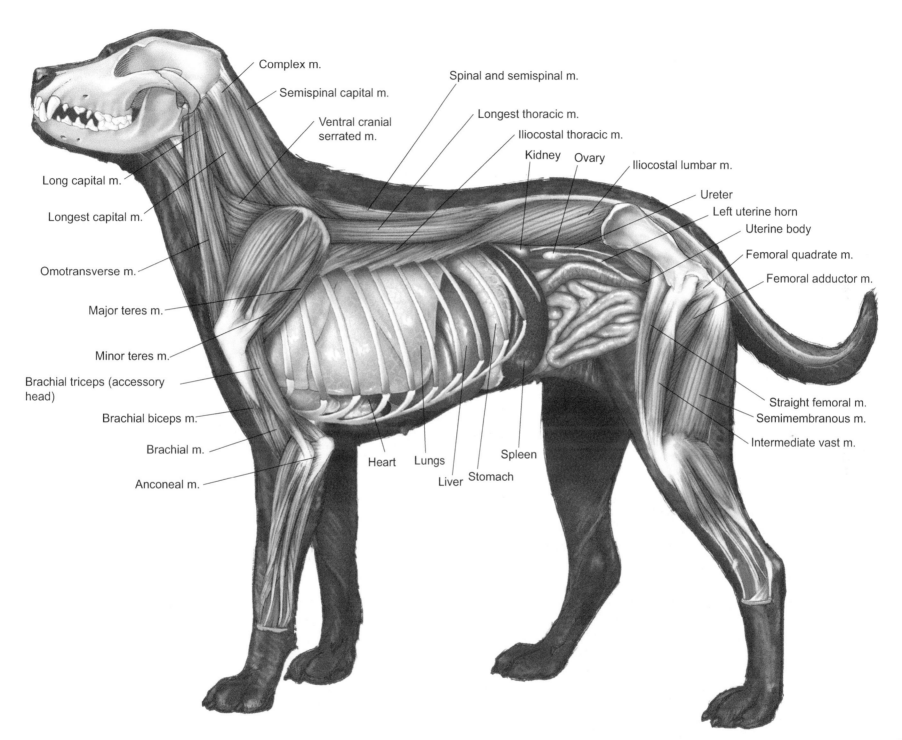

Complex m.

Semispinal capital m.

Ventral cranial
serrated m.

Spinal and semispinal m.

Longest thoracic m.

Iliocostal thoracic m.

Kidney   Ovary

Iliocostal lumbar m.

Ureter

Left uterine horn

Uterine body

Femoral quadrate m.

Femoral adductor m.

Long capital m.

Longest capital m.

Omotransverse m.

Major teres m.

Minor teres m.

Brachial triceps (accessory
head)

Brachial biceps m.

Brachial m.

Anconeal m.

Heart   Lungs   Spleen

Liver   Stomach

Straight femoral m.

Semimembranous m.

Intermediate vast m.

PLATE 1.8 Deep cervical and back muscles (m.), major joints, and in situ viscera of the bitch.

9

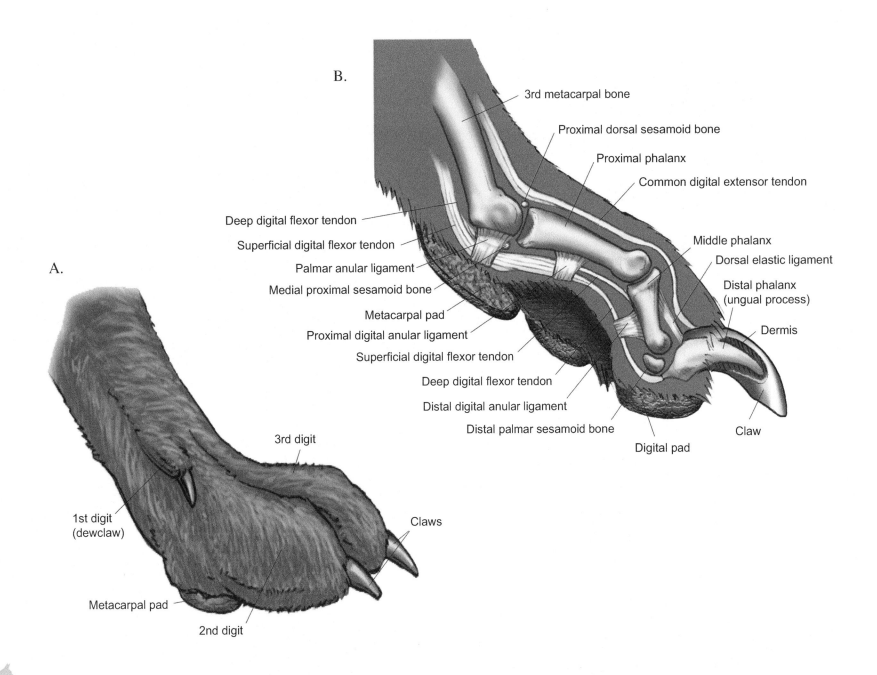

B.

3rd metacarpal bone

Proximal dorsal sesamoid bone

Proximal phalanx

Common digital extensor tendon

Deep digital flexor tendon

Superficial digital flexor tendon

Palmar anular ligament

Medial proximal sesamoid bone

Metacarpal pad

Proximal digital anular ligament

Superficial digital flexor tendon

Deep digital flexor tendon

Distal digital anular ligament

Distal palmar sesamoid bone

Middle phalanx

Dorsal elastic ligament

Distal phalanx (ungual process)

Dermis

Claw

Digital pad

A.

3rd digit

1st digit (dewclaw)

Claws

Metacarpal pad

2nd digit

PLATE 1.9 Forepaw: A. Medial superficial view, B. Medial deep view.

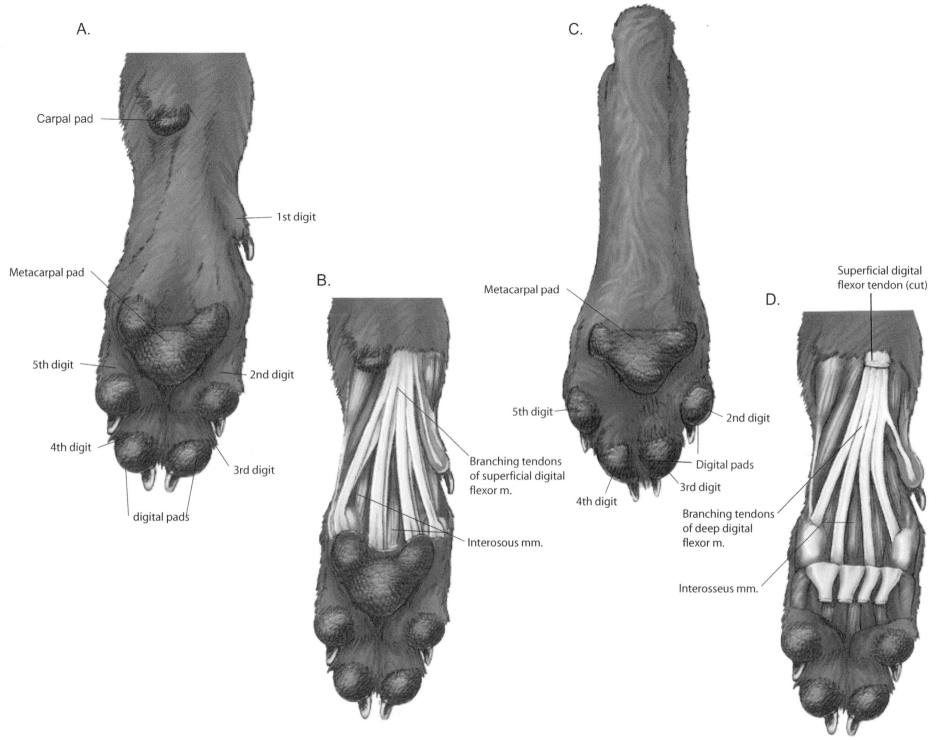

A.

Carpal pad

1st digit

Metacarpal pad

5th digit

2nd digit

4th digit

3rd digit

digital pads

B.

Branching tendons
of superficial digital
flexor m.

Interosous mm.

C.

Metacarpal pad

5th digit

2nd digit

Digital pads

3rd digit

4th digit

D.

Superficial digital
flexor tendon (cut)

Branching tendons
of deep digital
flexor m.

Interosseus mm.

PLATE 1.10 A. Palmar view of the forepaw; B. Palmar view of superficial dissection of forepaw;
C. Plantar view of hindpaw; D. Plantar view of superficial dissection of hindpaw.

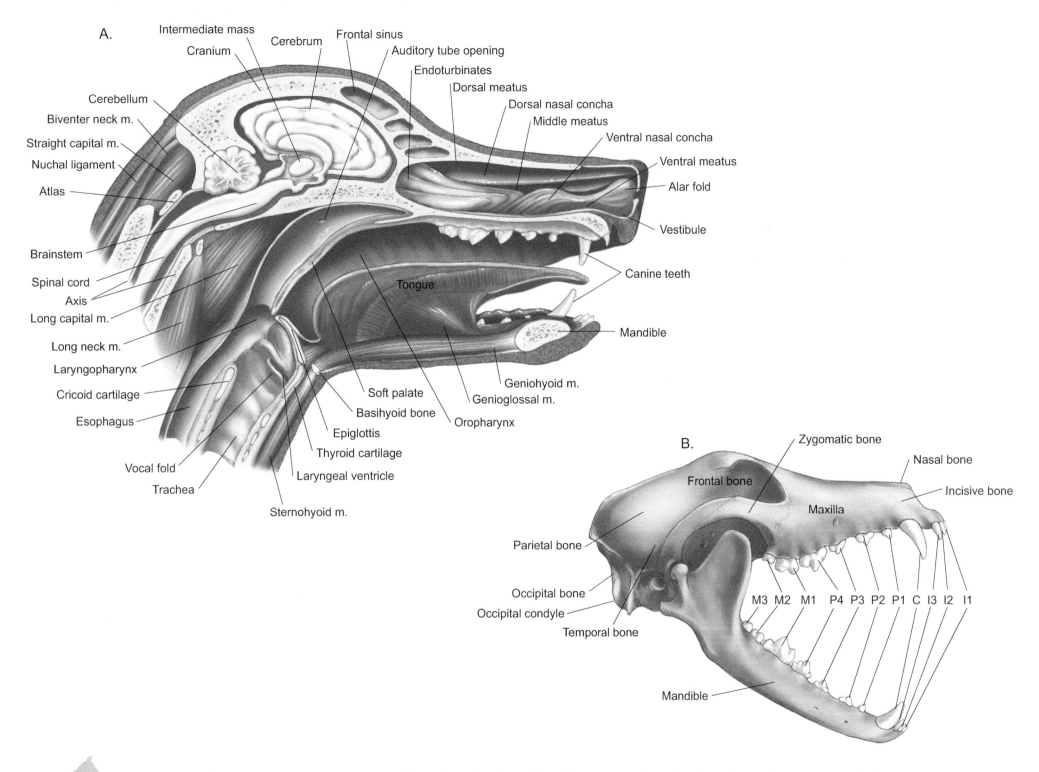

A.

Intermediate mass
Cranium
Cerebrum
Frontal sinus
Auditory tube opening
Endoturbinates
Dorsal meatus
Dorsal nasal concha
Middle meatus
Ventral nasal concha
Ventral meatus
Alar fold
Vestibule

Cerebellum
Biventer neck m.
Straight capital m.
Nuchal ligament
Atlas
Brainstem
Spinal cord
Axis
Long capital m.
Long neck m.
Laryngopharynx
Cricoid cartilage
Esophagus
Vocal fold
Trachea
Sternohyoid m.
Epiglottis
Thyroid cartilage
Laryngeal ventricle
Basihyoid bone
Soft palate
Oropharynx
Geniohyoid m.
Genioglossal m.
Mandible
Canine teeth
Tongue

B.

Frontal bone
Zygomatic bone
Nasal bone
Maxilla
Incisive bone
Parietal bone
Occipital bone
Occipital condyle
Temporal bone
Mandible
M3 M2 M1 P4 P3 P2 P1 C I3 I2 I1

12   PLATE 1.11 A. Medial sagittal section of head. B. Skull and dentition (M- molar, I- incisor, C - canine, P - premolar).

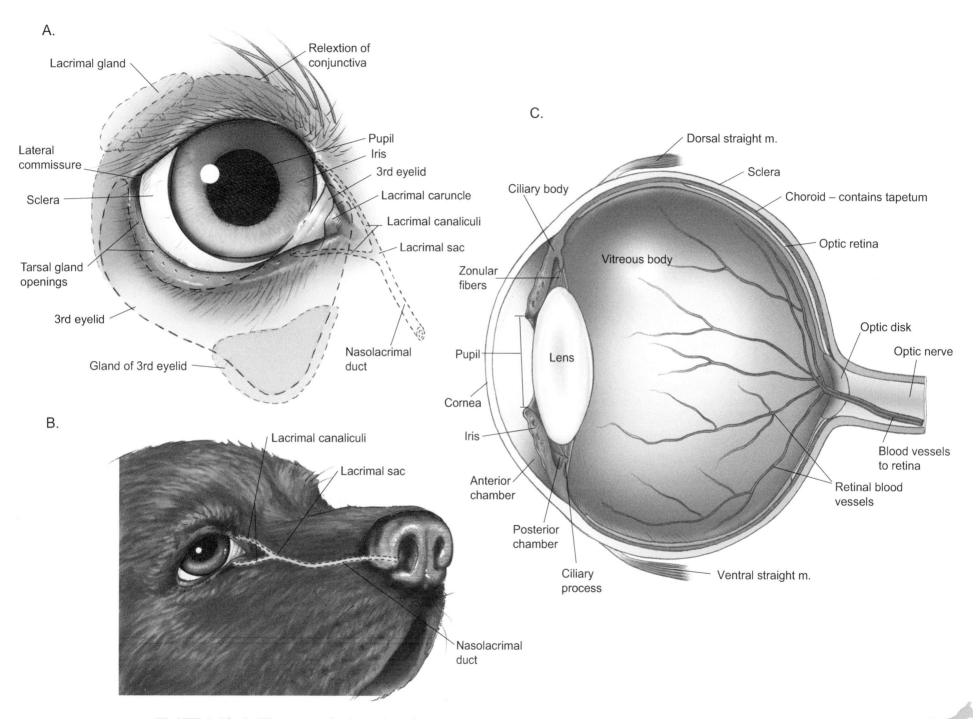

A.

Lacrimal gland

Relextion of conjunctiva

Lateral commissure

Sclera

Tarsal gland openings

3rd eyelid

Gland of 3rd eyelid

Pupil

Iris

3rd eyelid

Lacrimal caruncle

Lacrimal canaliculi

Lacrimal sac

Nasolacrimal duct

B.

Lacrimal canaliculi

Lacrimal sac

Nasolacrimal duct

C.

Dorsal straight m.

Sclera

Choroid – contains tapetum

Optic retina

Ciliary body

Vitreous body

Optic disk

Zonular fibers

Optic nerve

Pupil

Lens

Cornea

Iris

Blood vessels to retina

Anterior chamber

Retinal blood vessels

Posterior chamber

Ciliary process

Ventral straight m.

PLATE 1.12 A. The eye and adnexal ocular structures. B. Nasolacrimal duct. C. Median section of eye.

13

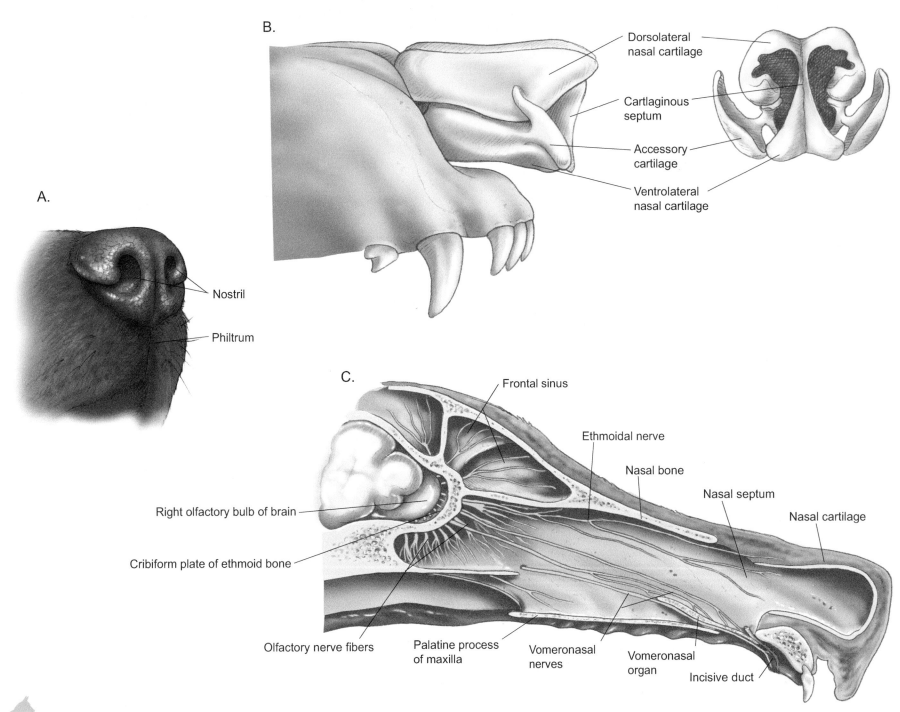

A.

B.

Dorsolateral
nasal cartilage

Cartlaginous
septum

Accessory
cartilage

Ventrolateral
nasal cartilage

Nostril

Philtrum

C.

Frontal sinus

Ethmoidal nerve

Nasal bone

Nasal septum

Nasal cartilage

Right olfactory bulb of brain

Cribiform plate of ethmoid bone

Olfactory nerve fibers

Palatine process
of maxilla

Vomeronasal
nerves

Vomeronasal
organ

Incisive duct

PLATE 1.13 Rt. nasal fossa. A. External nares. B. Nasal cartilages. C. Medial sagittal section of the muzzle.

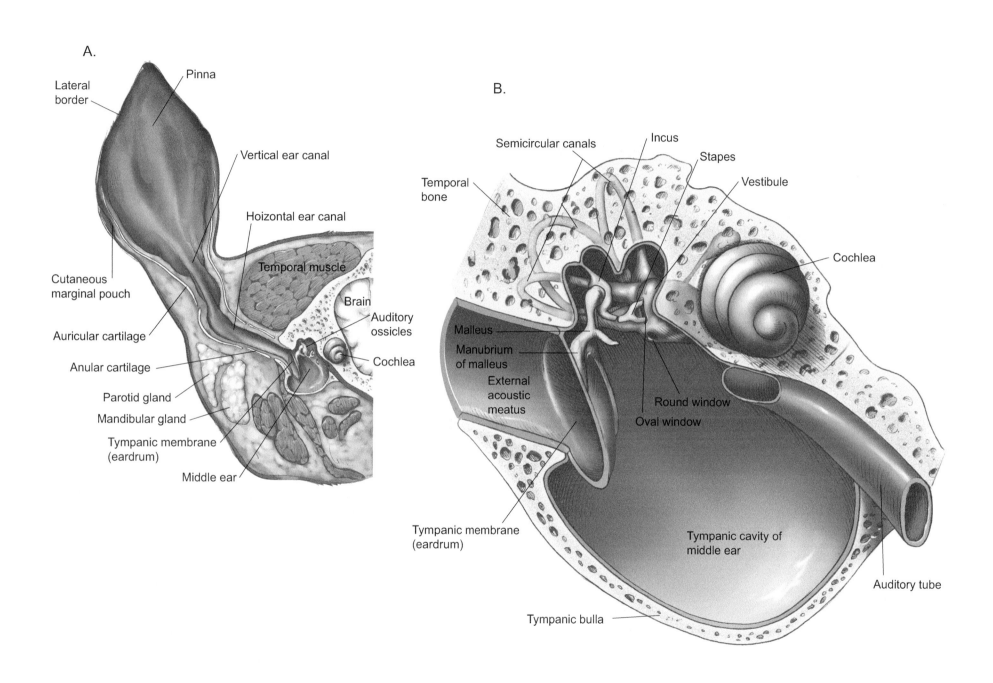

A.

Lateral border

Pinna

Vertical ear canal

Hoizontal ear canal

Temporal muscle

Brain

Cutaneous marginal pouch

Auricular cartilage

Anular cartilage

Parotid gland

Mandibular gland

Tympanic membrane (eardrum)

Middle ear

Auditory ossicles

Cochlea

B.

Semicircular canals

Incus

Stapes

Vestibule

Temporal bone

Cochlea

Malleus

Manubrium of malleus

External acoustic meatus

Round window

Oval window

Tympanic membrane (eardrum)

Tympanic cavity of middle ear

Auditory tube

Tympanic bulla

PLATE 1.14 The ear. A. Coronal section of the head and external ear. B. Middle and inner ear.

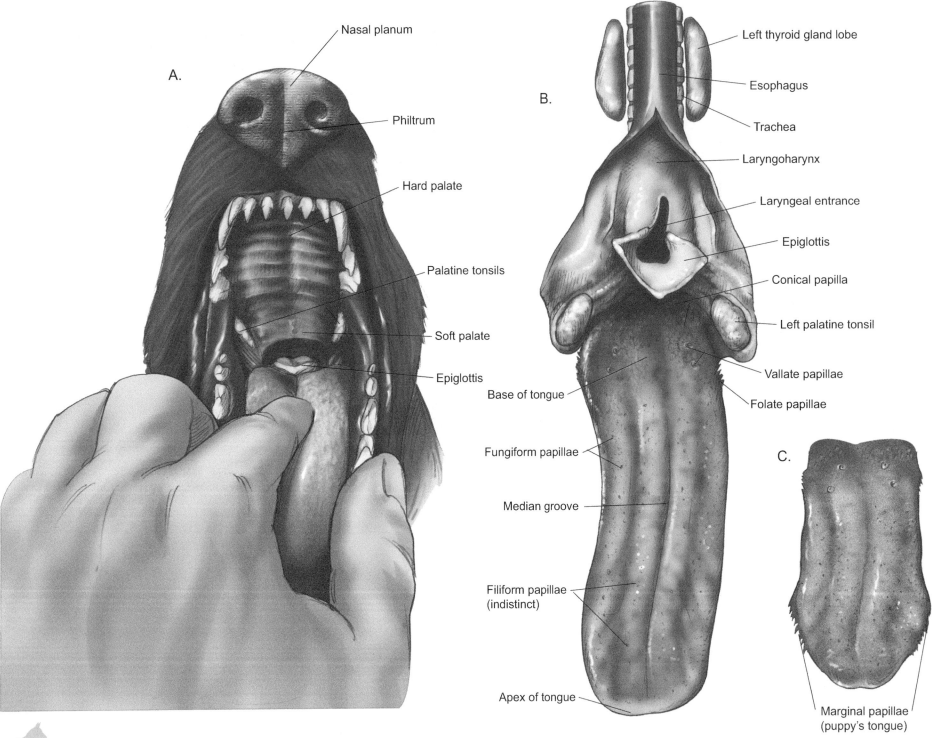

A.

Nasal planum

Philtrum

Hard palate

Palatine tonsils

Soft palate

Epiglottis

B.

Left thyroid gland lobe

Esophagus

Trachea

Laryngoharynx

Laryngeal entrance

Epiglottis

Conical papilla

Left palatine tonsil

Vallate papillae

Folate papillae

Base of tongue

Fungiform papillae

Median groove

Filiform papillae
(indistinct)

Apex of tongue

C.

Marginal papillae
(puppy's tongue)

16

PLATE 1.15 Oral cavity, tongue, and esophagus

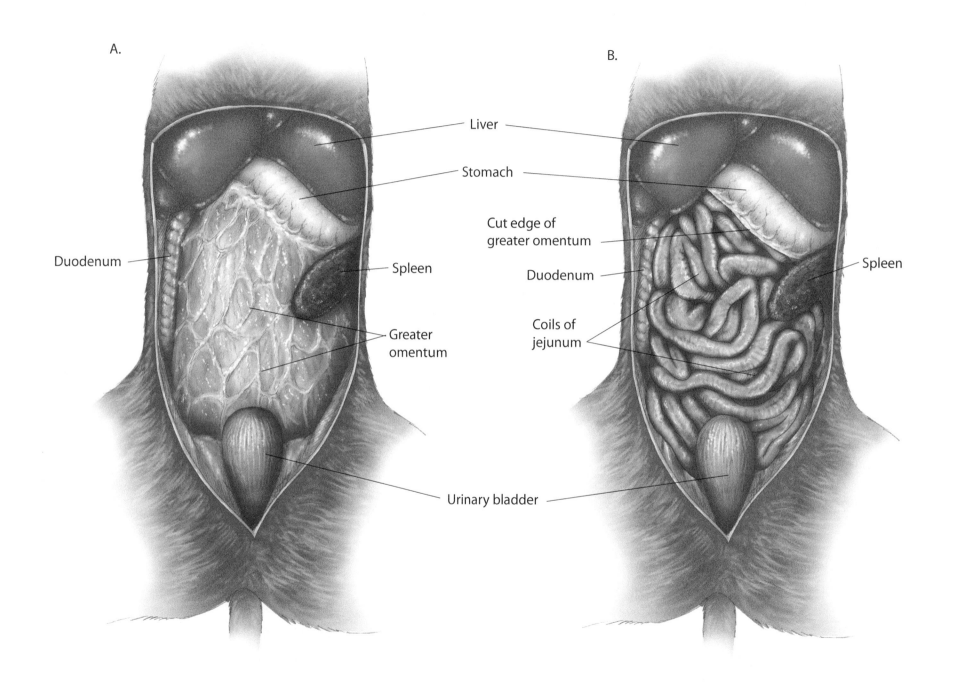

A.

B.

Liver

Stomach

Cut edge of
greater omentum

Duodenum

Spleen

Duodenum

Spleen

Greater
omentum

Coils of
jejunum

Urinary bladder

PLATE 1.16 A. Ventral view of dog abdomen with abdominal wall removed. B. View with greater omentum removed.

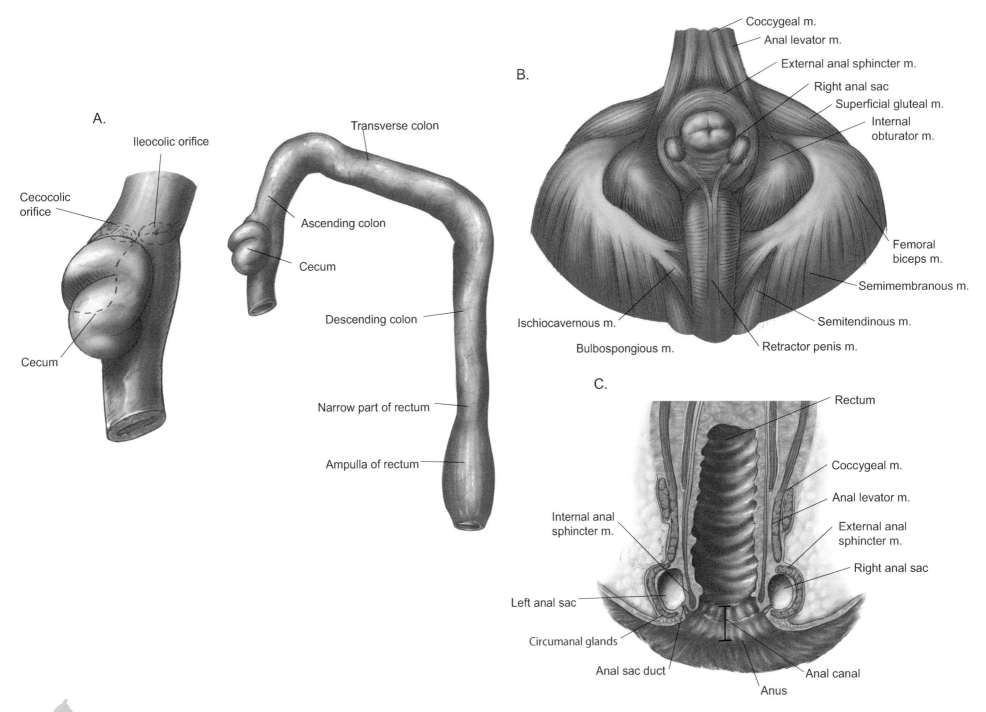

A. Large intestine.

Ileocolic orifice

Cecocolic orifice

Cecum

Cecum

Transverse colon

Ascending colon

Cecum

Descending colon

Narrow part of rectum

Ampulla of rectum

B.

Coccygeal m.

Anal levator m.

External anal sphincter m.

Right anal sac

Superficial gluteal m.

Internal obturator m.

Femoral biceps m.

Semimembranous m.

Semitendinous m.

Retractor penis m.

Bulbospongious m.

Ischiocavernous m.

C.

Rectum

Coccygeal m.

Anal levator m.

External anal sphincter m.

Right anal sac

Anal canal

Anus

Anal sac duct

Circumanal glands

Left anal sac

Internal anal sphincter m.

18   PLATE 1.17 A. Large intestine. B. Superficial view of anus and anal sacs. C. Dorsal section of rectum, anus, and anal sacs.

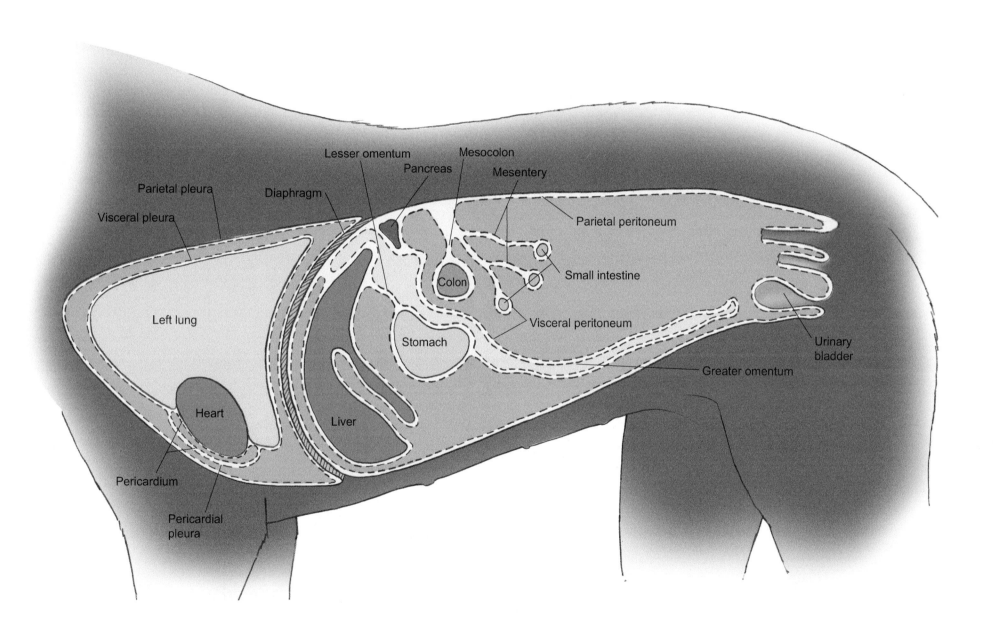

PLATE 1.18 Body cavities and serous membranes.

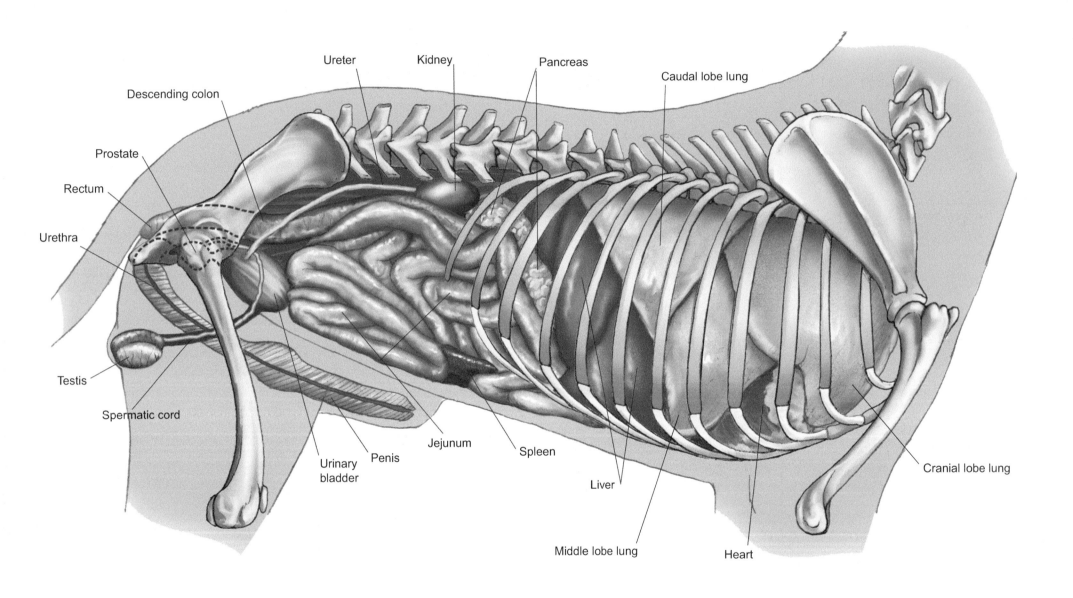

Ureter   Kidney   Pancreas

Caudal lobe lung

Descending colon

Prostate

Rectum

Urethra

Testis

Spermatic cord

Urinary bladder   Penis   Jejunum   Spleen

Liver

Middle lobe lung   Heart

Cranial lobe lung

PLATE 1.19 Thoracic, abdominal, and pelvic viscera related to the skeleton of the dog. Right lateral view.

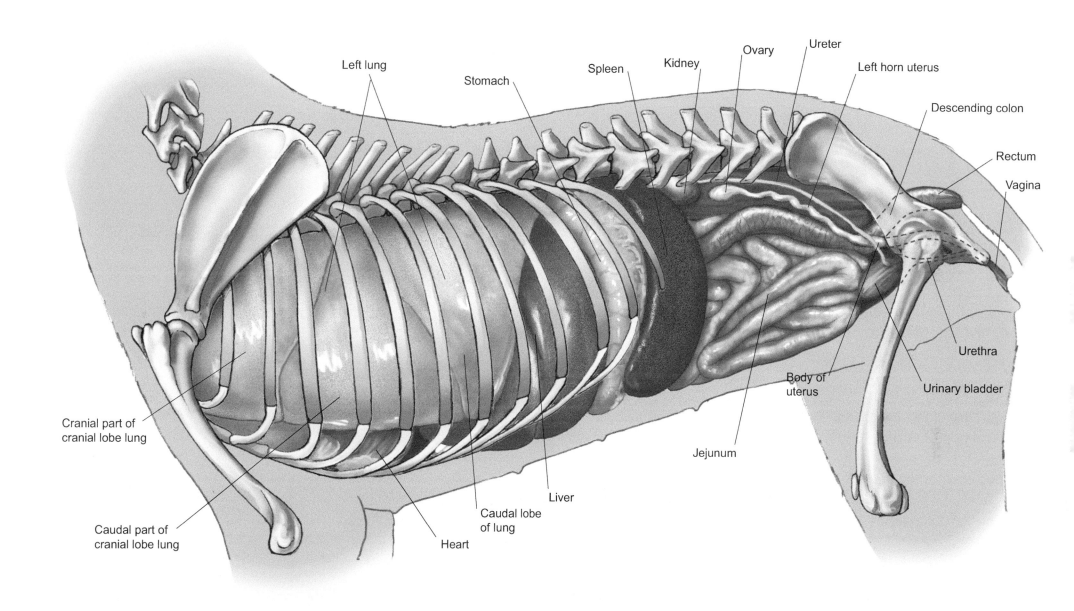

Left lung

Stomach

Spleen

Kidney

Ovary

Ureter

Left horn uterus

Descending colon

Rectum

Vagina

Cranial part of
cranial lobe lung

Caudal part of
cranial lobe lung

Heart

Caudal lobe
of lung

Liver

Jejunum

Body of
uterus

Urethra

Urinary bladder

PLATE 1.20 Thoracic, abdominal, and pelvic viscera related to the skeleton of the bitch. Left lateral view.

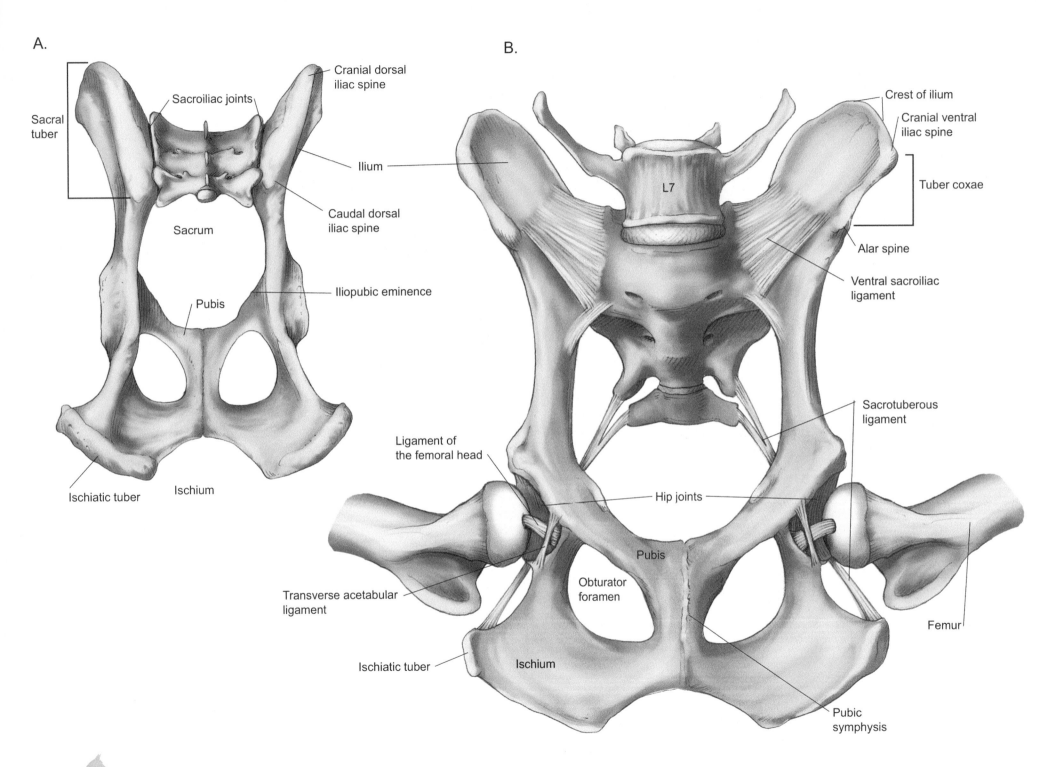

A.

Sacral tuber

Sacroiliac joints

Cranial dorsal iliac spine

Sacrum

Ilium

Caudal dorsal iliac spine

Pubis

Iliopubic eminence

Ischiatic tuber

Ischium

B.

Crest of ilium

Cranial ventral iliac spine

L7

Ilium

Tuber coxae

Alar spine

Ventral sacroiliac ligament

Sacrotuberous ligament

Ligament of the femoral head

Hip joints

Transverse acetabular ligament

Pubis

Obturator foramen

Femur

Ischiatic tuber

Ischium

Pubic symphysis

22

PLATE 1.21 Pelvis and hip joint: A. Dorsal view, B. Ventral view.

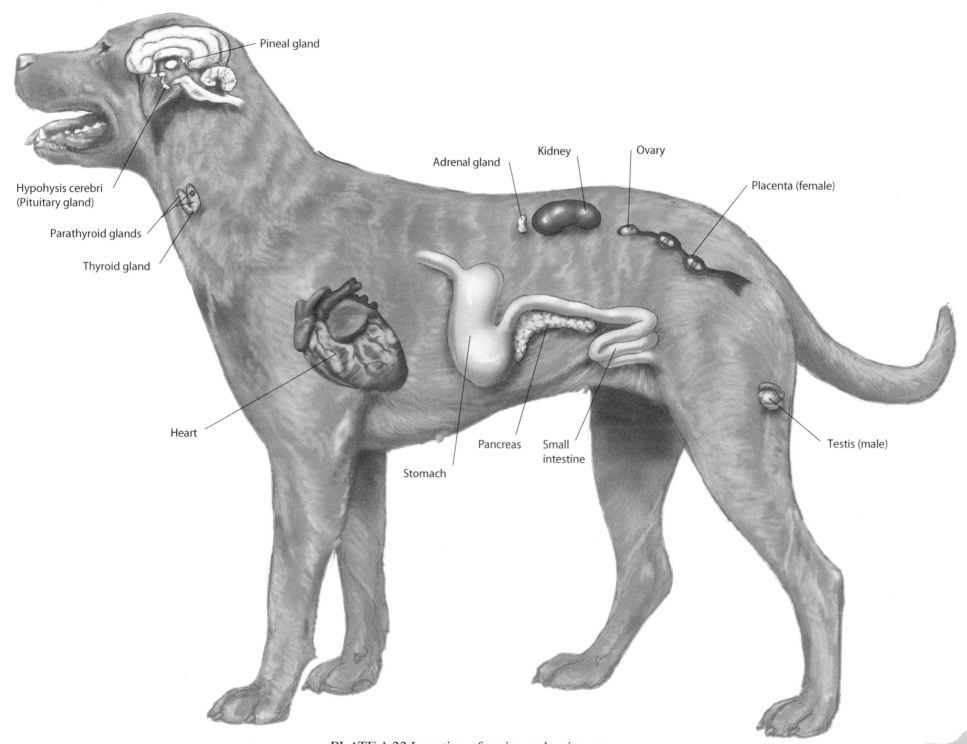

Pineal gland

Hypohysis cerebri
(Pituitary gland)

Parathyroid glands

Thyroid gland

Heart

Adrenal gland

Kidney

Ovary

Placenta (female)

Stomach

Pancreas

Small
intestine

Testis (male)

PLATE 1.22 Location of major endocrine organs.

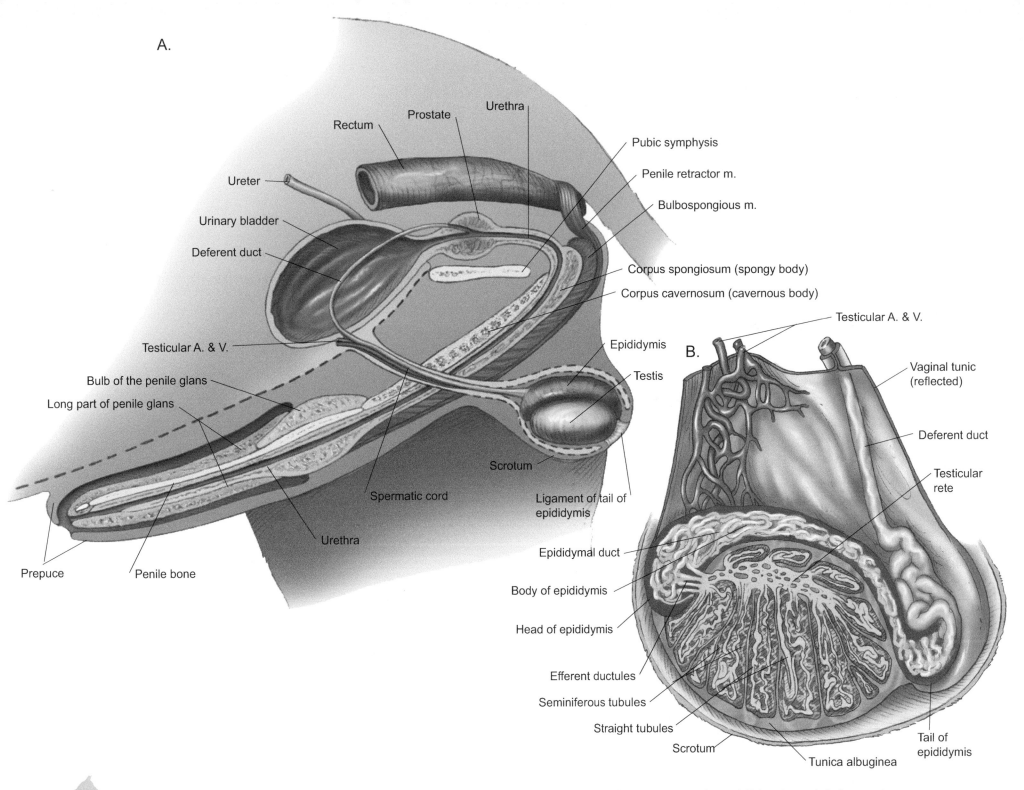

A.

Rectum

Prostate

Urethra

Pubic symphysis

Penile retractor m.

Bulbospongious m.

Ureter

Urinary bladder

Deferent duct

Corpus spongiosum (spongy body)

Corpus cavernosum (cavernous body)

Testicular A. & V.

Epididymis

Testis

Bulb of the penile glans

Long part of penile glans

Scrotum

Spermatic cord

Ligament of tail of epididymis

Urethra

Prepuce

Penile bone

B.

Testicular A. & V.

Vaginal tunic (reflected)

Deferent duct

Testicular rete

Epididymal duct

Body of epididymis

Head of epididymis

Efferent ductules

Seminiferous tubules

Straight tubules

Scrotum

Tunica albuginea

Tail of epididymis

24   PLATE 1.23 Relations of the reproductive organs of the dog: A. Left sagittal view, B. Testis, epididymis and deferent duct.

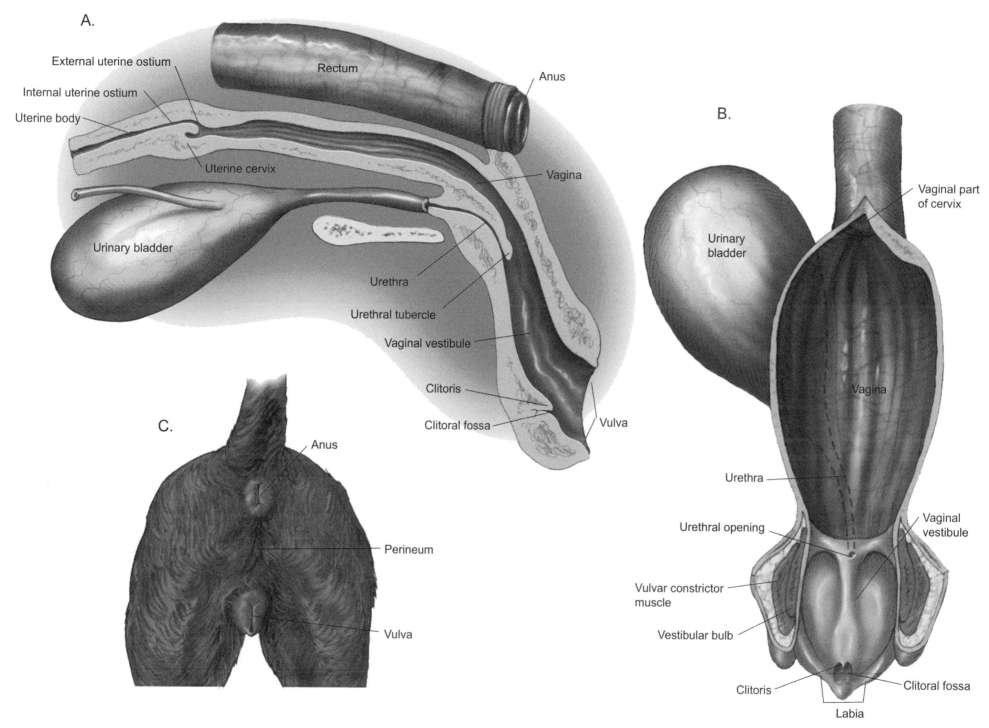

A.

External uterine ostium

Internal uterine ostium

Uterine body

Rectum

Anus

Uterine cervix

Vagina

Urinary bladder

Urethra

Urethral tubercle

Vaginal vestibule

Clitoris

Clitoral fossa

Vulva

B.

Vaginal part of cervix

Urinary bladder

Vagina

Urethra

Urethral opening

Vaginal vestibule

Vulvar constrictor muscle

Vestibular bulb

Clitoris

Clitoral fossa

Labia

C.

Anus

Perineum

Vulva

PLATE 1.24 Relations of the reproductive organs of the bitch: A. Sagittal section of uterine cervix, vagina and vulva, B. Dorsal view of female genitalia, C. Caudal view of a female.

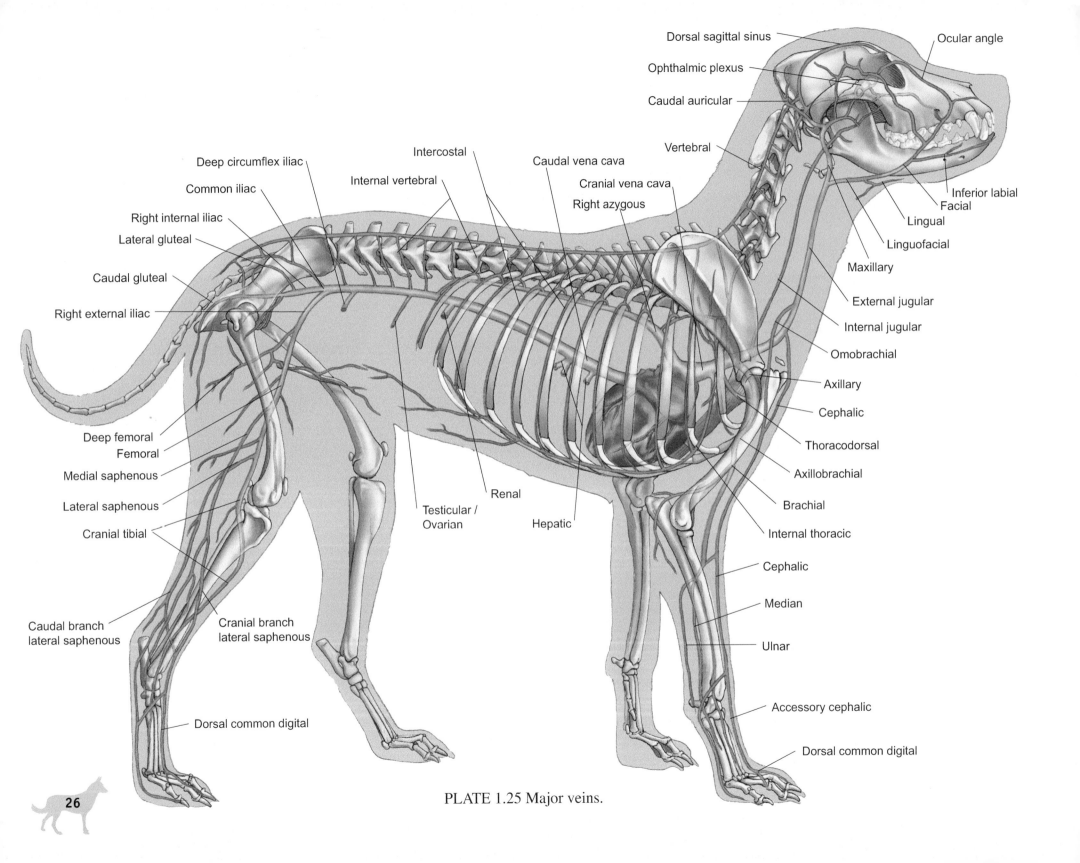

Dorsal sagittal sinus

Ocular angle

Ophthalmic plexus

Caudal auricular

Vertebral

Inferior labial

Facial

Intercostal

Caudal vena cava

Lingual

Deep circumflex iliac

Internal vertebral

Cranial vena cava

Linguofacial

Common iliac

Right azygous

Maxillary

Right internal iliac

Lateral gluteal

External jugular

Caudal gluteal

Internal jugular

Right external iliac

Omobrachial

Axillary

Cephalic

Deep femoral

Thoracodorsal

Femoral

Axillobrachial

Medial saphenous

Renal

Brachial

Lateral saphenous

Testicular /
Ovarian

Hepatic

Internal thoracic

Cranial tibial

Cephalic

Median

Cranial branch
lateral saphenous

Ulnar

Caudal branch
lateral saphenous

Accessory cephalic

Dorsal common digital

Dorsal common digital

26

PLATE 1.25 Major veins.

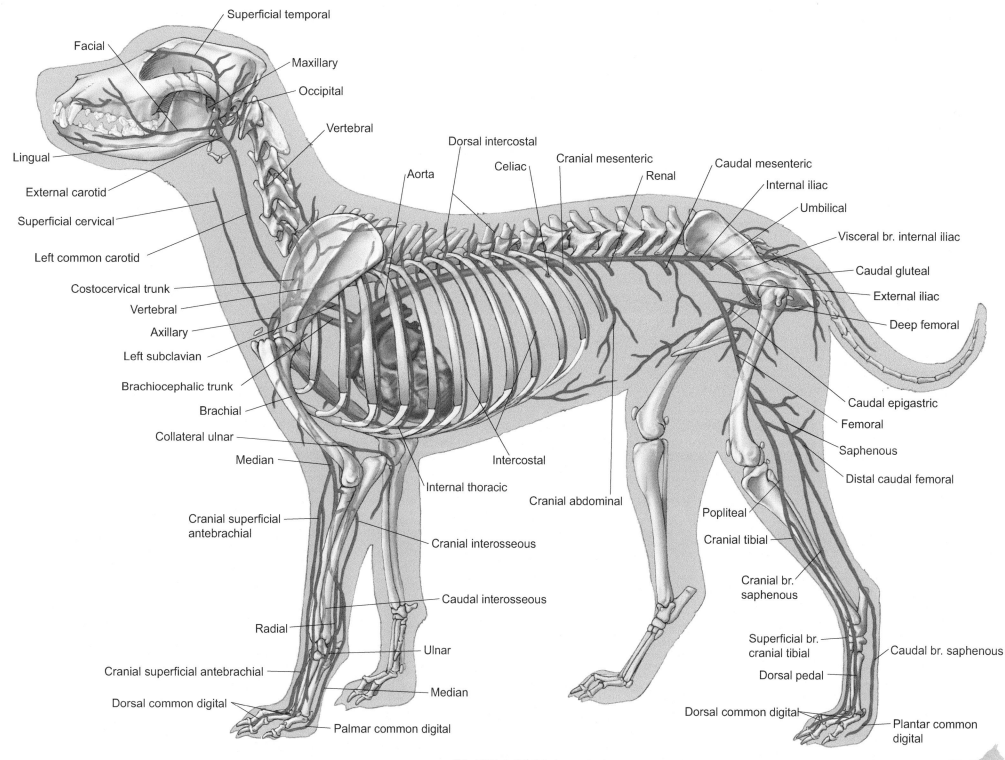

PLATE 1.26 Major arteries.

27

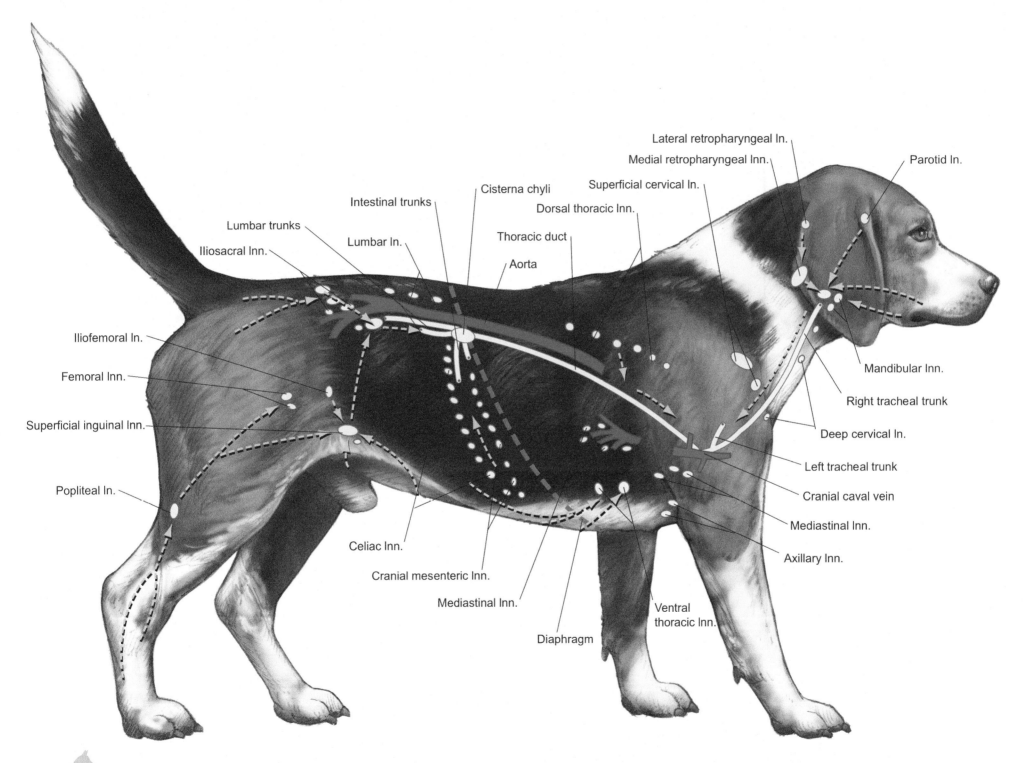

Lateral retropharyngeal ln.

Medial retropharyngeal lnn.

Parotid ln.

Superficial cervical ln.

Cisterna chyli

Dorsal thoracic lnn.

Intestinal trunks

Lumbar trunks

Lumbar ln.

Thoracic duct

Iliosacral lnn.

Aorta

Iliofemoral ln.

Mandibular lnn.

Femoral lnn.

Right tracheal trunk

Superficial inguinal lnn.

Deep cervical ln.

Left tracheal trunk

Popliteal ln.

Cranial caval vein

Mediastinal lnn.

Celiac lnn.

Axillary lnn.

Cranial mesenteric lnn.

Mediastinal lnn.

Ventral
thoracic lnn.

Diaphragm

PLATE 1.27 Lymph nodes (lnn.) and vessels.

28

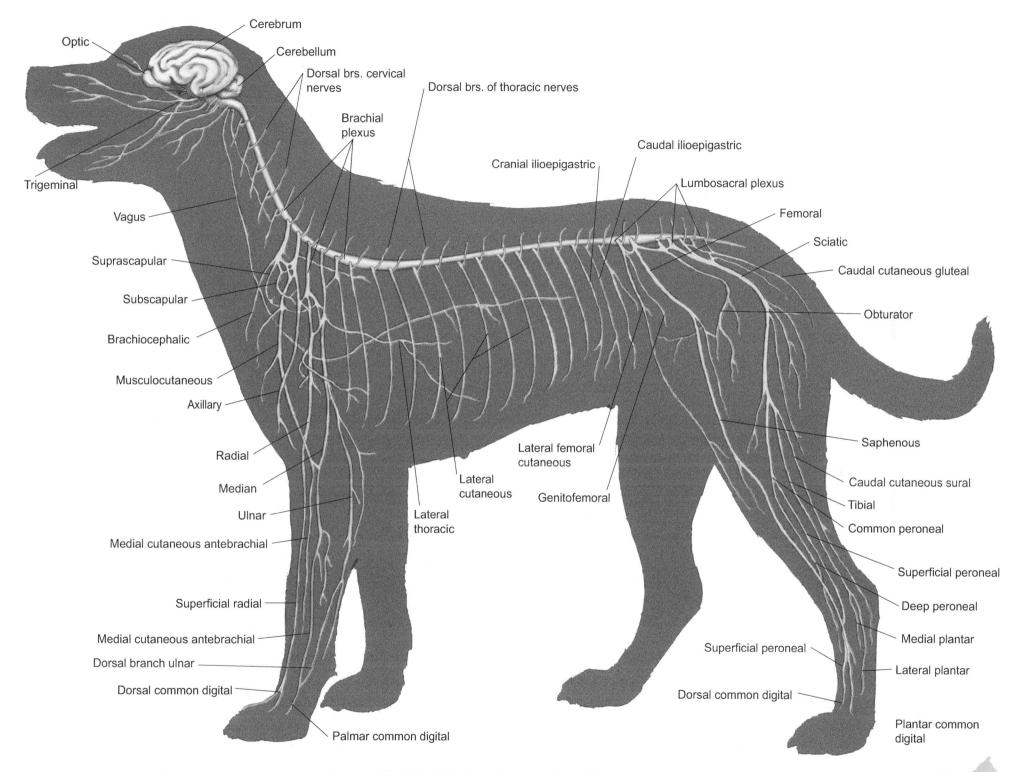

PLATE 1.28 Central and peripheral nervous systems.

29

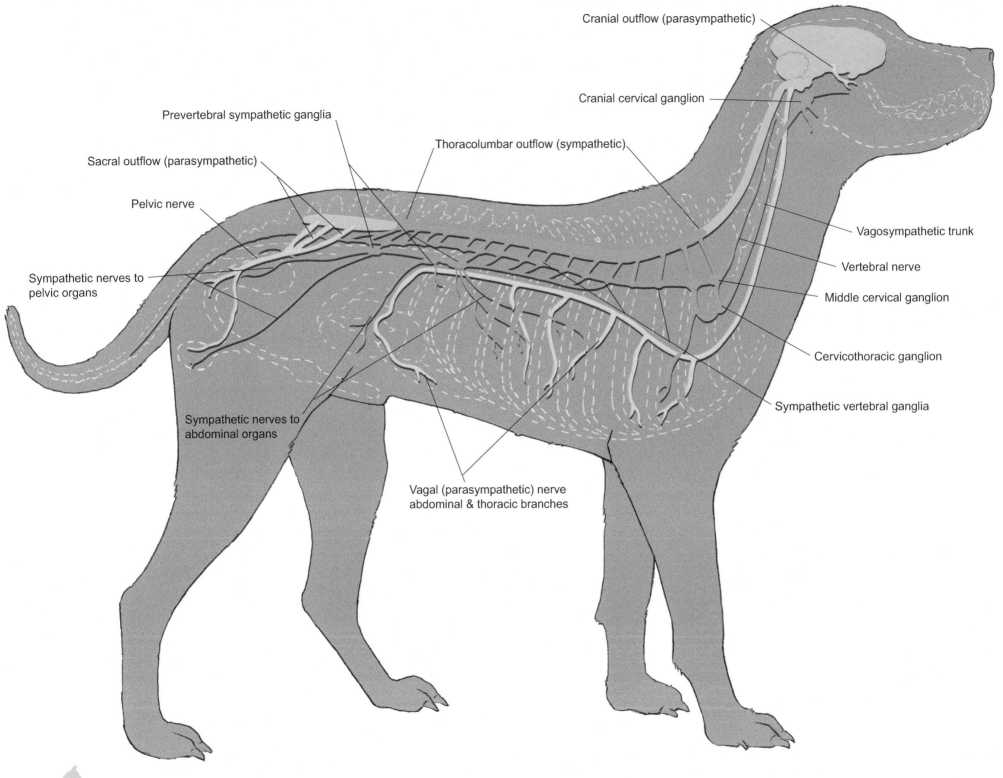

Cranial outflow (parasympathetic)

Cranial cervical ganglion

Prevertebral sympathetic ganglia

Thoracolumbar outflow (sympathetic)

Sacral outflow (parasympathetic)

Pelvic nerve

Vagosympathetic trunk

Vertebral nerve

Sympathetic nerves to pelvic organs

Middle cervical ganglion

Cervicothoracic ganglion

Sympathetic nerves to abdominal organs

Sympathetic vertebral ganglia

Vagal (parasympathetic) nerve abdominal & thoracic branches

PLATE 1.29 Autonomic nervous system: Sym. = Sympathetic division and Para. = Parasympathetic division.

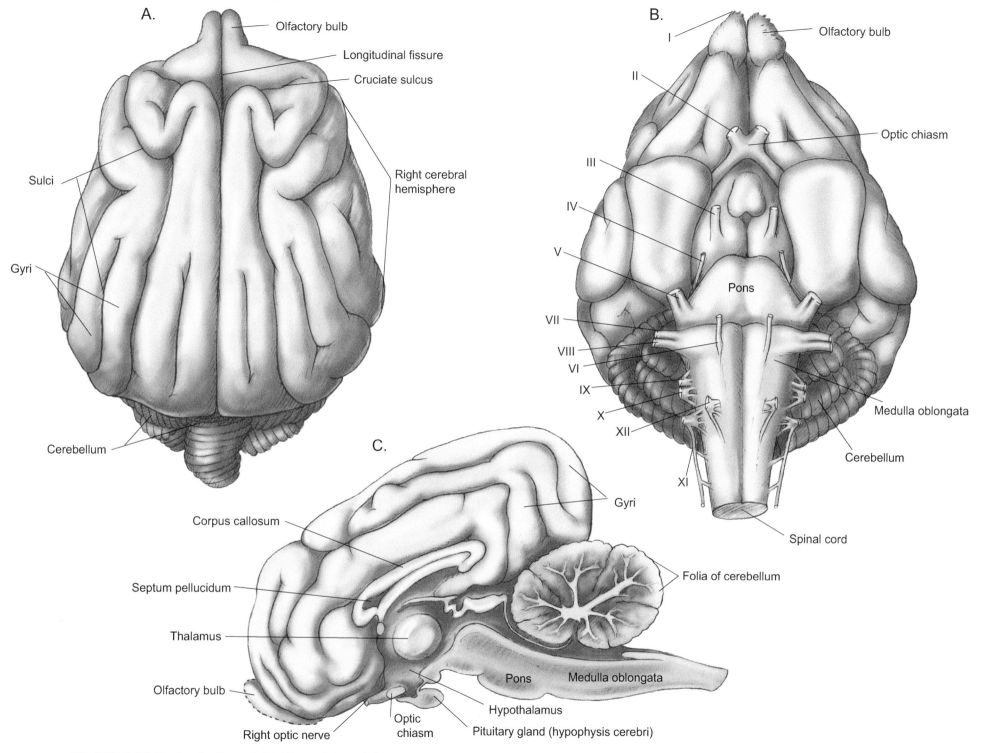

A.

Olfactory bulb

Longitudinal fissure

Cruciate sulcus

Right cerebral hemisphere

Sulci

Gyri

Cerebellum

B.

I

Olfactory bulb

II

Optic chiasm

III

IV

V

Pons

VII

VIII

VI

IX

X

XII

Medulla oblongata

Cerebellum

XI

Spinal cord

C.

Gyri

Corpus callosum

Folia of cerebellum

Septum pellucidum

Thalamus

Pons

Medulla oblongata

Olfactory bulb

Hypothalamus

Right optic nerve

Optic chiasm

Pituitary gland (hypophysis cerebri)

PLATE 1.30 Brain: A. Dorsal, B. Ventral (cranial nerves I-XII), and C. Midsagittal views. I-olfactory, II-optic, III-oculomotor, IV-trochlear, V-trigeminal, VI-abducens, VII-facial, VIII-vestibulocochlear, IX-glossopharyngeal, X-vagus, XI-accessory, XII-hypoglossal nerves.

SECTION 2 THE CAT

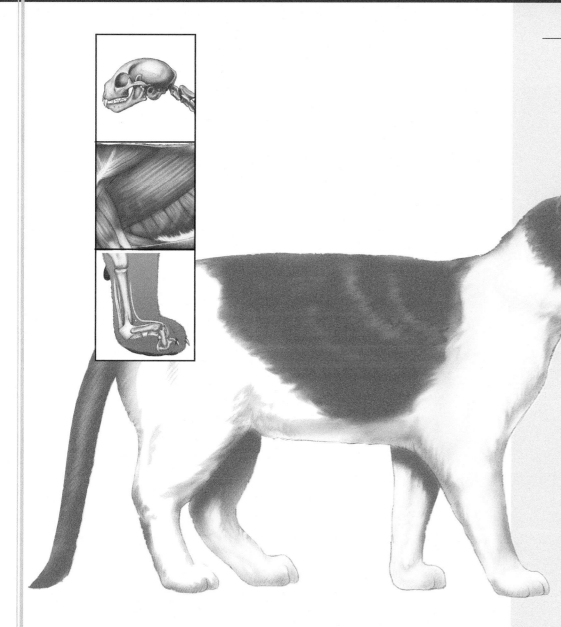

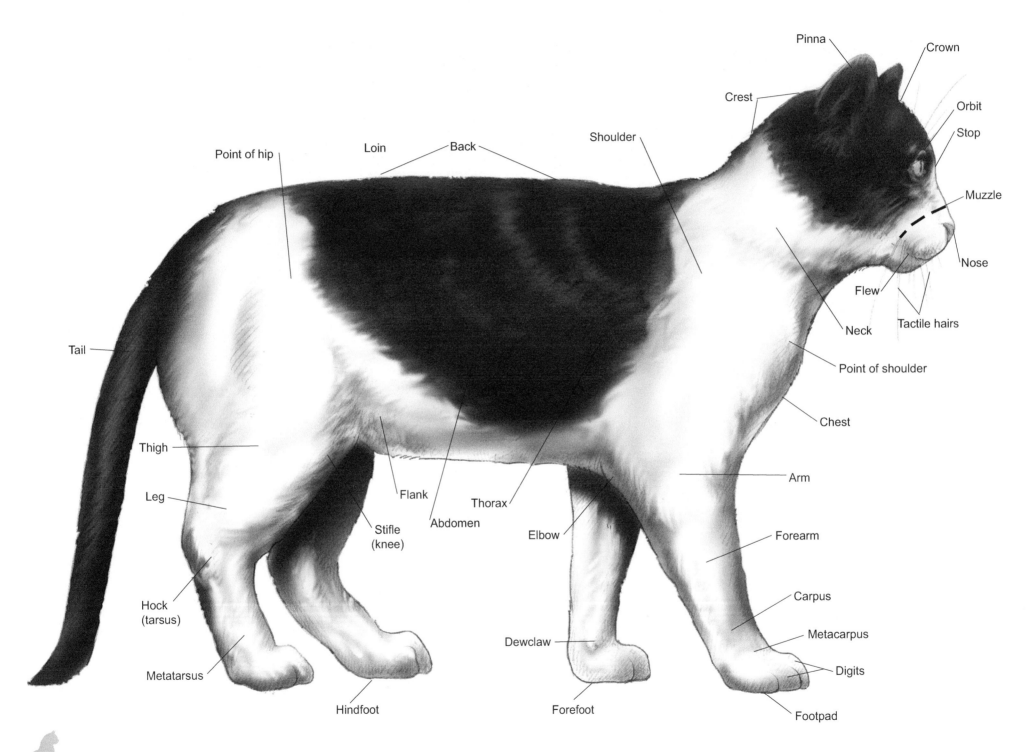

PLATE 2.1 Lateral view of the male cat (Domestic Shorthair).

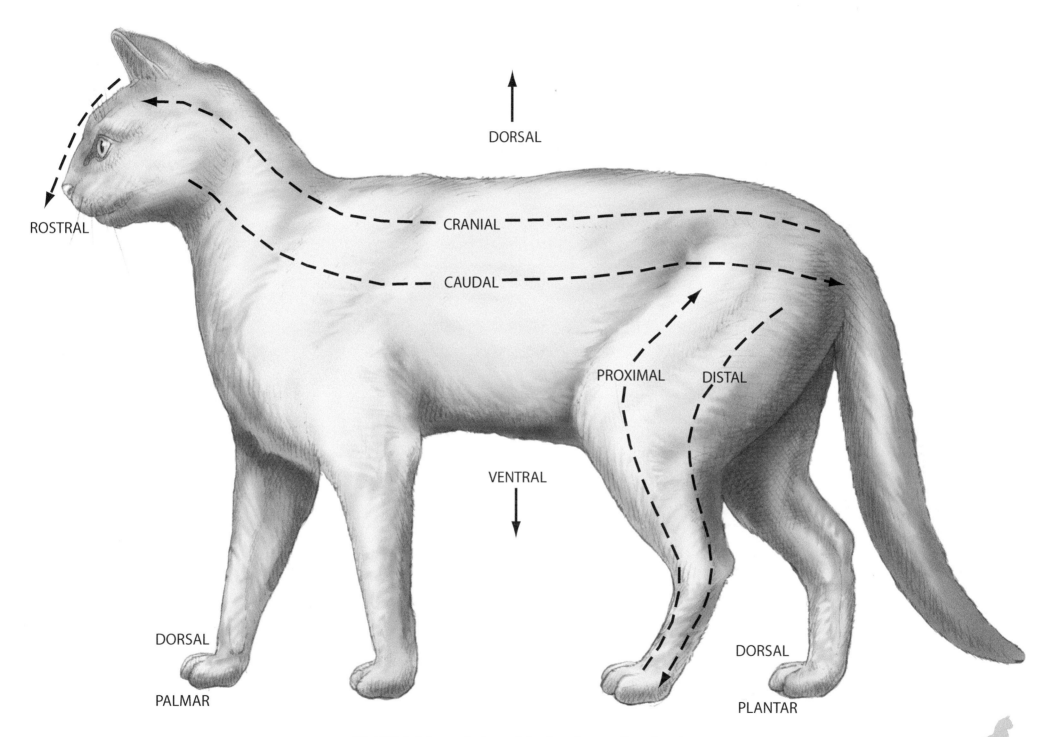

DORSAL

ROSTRAL

CRANIAL

CAUDAL

PROXIMAL   DISTAL

VENTRAL

DORSAL

PALMAR

DORSAL

PLANTAR

PLATE 2.2 Lateral view of the female cat, directional terms.

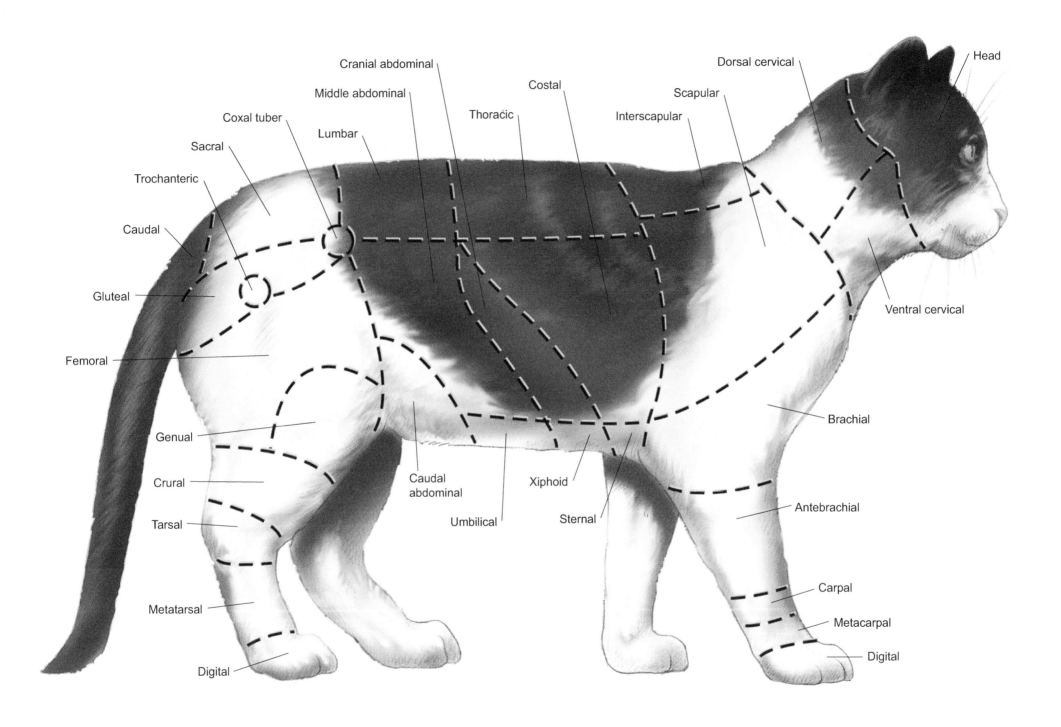

PLATE 2.3 Body regions.

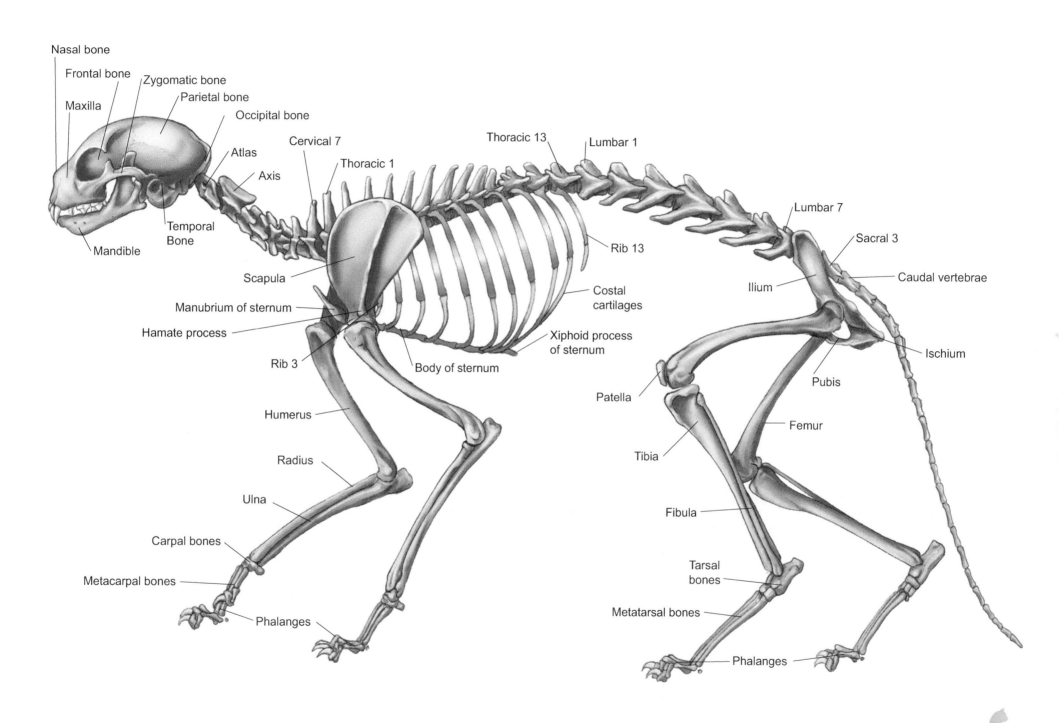

Nasal bone

Frontal bone

Zygomatic bone

Maxilla

Parietal bone

Occipital bone

Atlas

Axis

Cervical 7

Thoracic 1

Thoracic 13

Lumbar 1

Lumbar 7

Sacral 3

Caudal vertebrae

Temporal Bone

Mandible

Scapula

Rib 13

Ilium

Manubrium of sternum

Costal cartilages

Ischium

Hamate process

Xiphoid process of sternum

Pubis

Rib 3

Body of sternum

Patella

Humerus

Femur

Radius

Tibia

Ulna

Fibula

Carpal bones

Tarsal bones

Metacarpal bones

Metatarsal bones

Phalanges

Phalanges

PLATE 2.4 Skeleton.

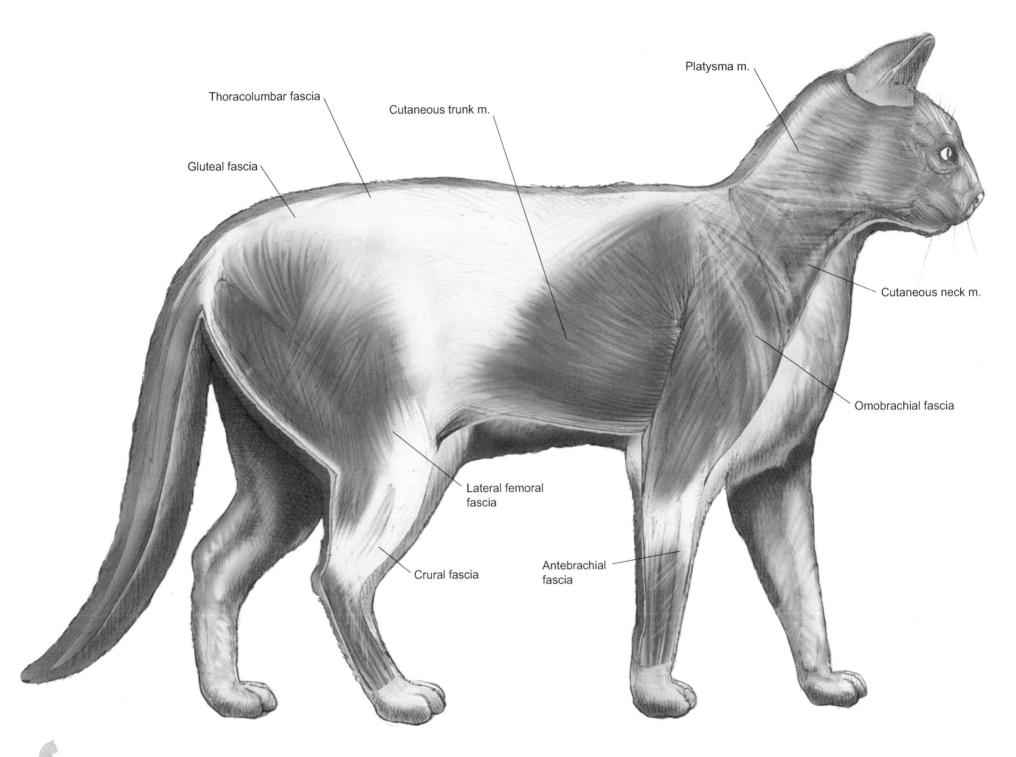

Thoracolumbar fascia

Cutaneous trunk m.

Platysma m.

Gluteal fascia

Cutaneous neck m.

Omobrachial fascia

Lateral femoral
fascia

Crural fascia

Antebrachial
fascia

38

PLATE 2.5 Cutaneous muscles and major fasciae of the male.

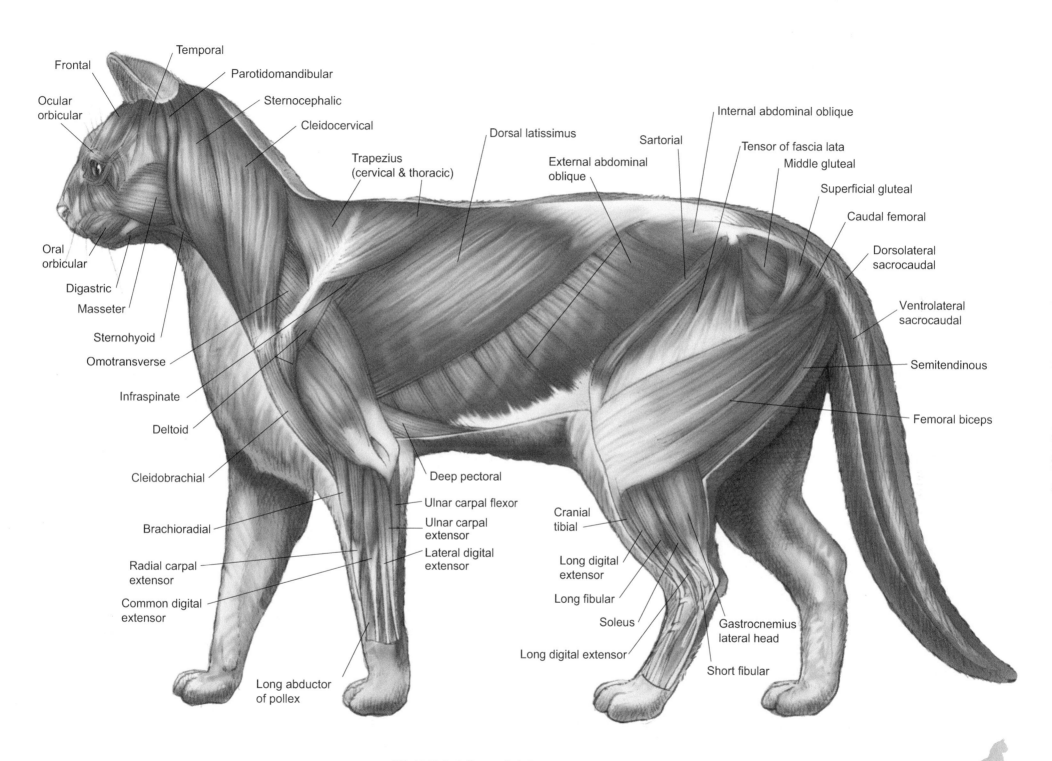

Frontal

Temporal

Ocular
orbicular

Parotidomandibular

Sternocephalic

Cleidocervical

Internal abdominal oblique

Dorsal latissimus

Sartorial

Tensor of fascia lata

Trapezius
(cervical & thoracic)

External abdominal
oblique

Middle gluteal

Superficial gluteal

Oral
orbicular

Caudal femoral

Dorsolateral
sacrocaudal

Digastric

Masseter

Ventrolateral
sacrocaudal

Sternohyoid

Omotransverse

Semitendinous

Infraspinate

Femoral biceps

Deltoid

Cleidobrachial

Deep pectoral

Brachioradial

Ulnar carpal flexor

Ulnar carpal
extensor

Cranial
tibial

Radial carpal
extensor

Lateral digital
extensor

Long digital
extensor

Common digital
extensor

Long fibular

Soleus

Long digital extensor

Gastrocnemius
lateral head

Long abductor
of pollex

Short fibular

PLATE 2.6 Superficial muscles (mm) of the female.

39

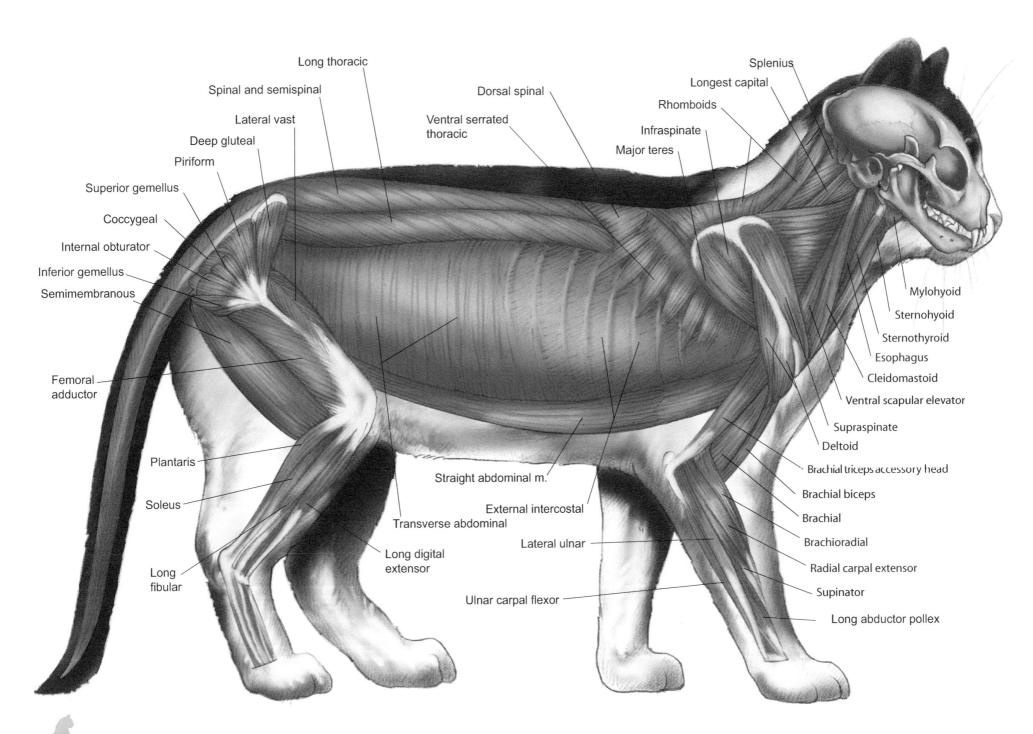

Long thoracic

Spinal and semispinal

Lateral vast

Deep gluteal

Piriform

Superior gemellus

Coccygeal

Internal obturator

Inferior gemellus

Semimembranous

Femoral adductor

Plantaris

Soleus

Long fibular

Long digital extensor

Transverse abdominal

Straight abdominal m.

External intercostal

Lateral ulnar

Ulnar carpal flexor

Dorsal spinal

Ventral serrated thoracic

Major teres

Splenius

Longest capital

Rhomboids

Infraspinate

Mylohyoid

Sternohyoid

Sternothyroid

Esophagus

Cleidomastoid

Ventral scapular elevator

Supraspinate

Deltoid

Brachial triceps accessory head

Brachial biceps

Brachial

Brachioradial

Radial carpal extensor

Supinator

Long abductor pollex

PLATE 2.7 Middle layer of muscles and in situ viscera of the male.

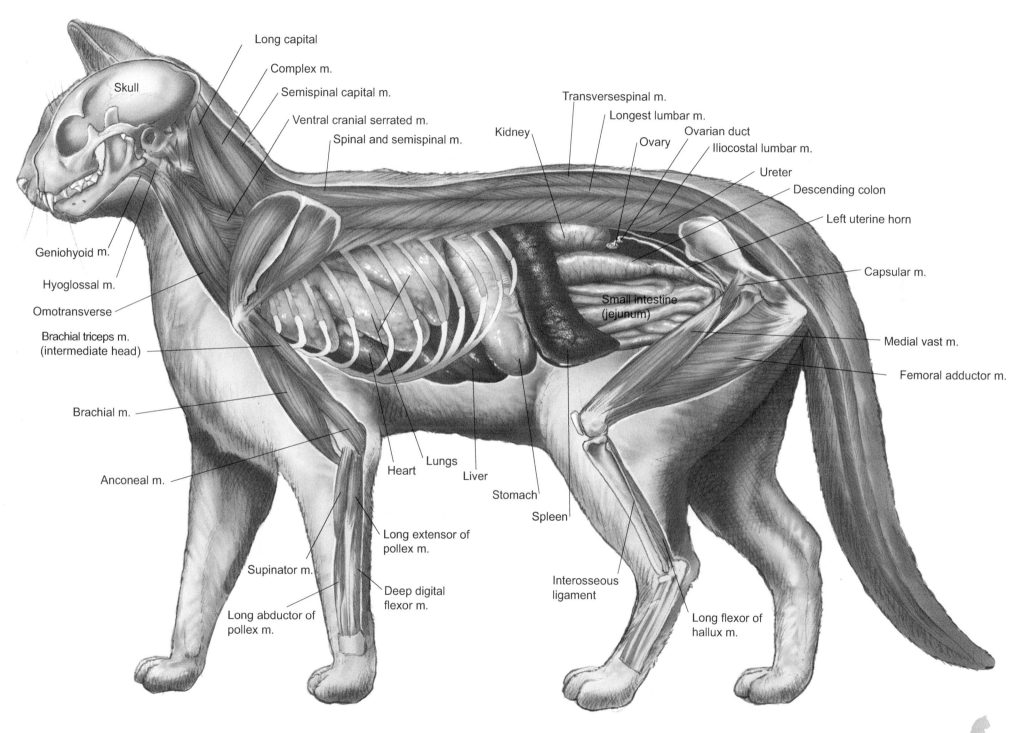

Long capital

Complex m.

Skull

Semispinal capital m.

Ventral cranial serrated m.

Spinal and semispinal m.

Kidney

Transversespinal m.

Longest lumbar m.

Ovary

Ovarian duct

Iliocostal lumbar m.

Ureter

Descending colon

Left uterine horn

Geniohyoid m.

Hyoglossal m.

Omotransverse

Brachial triceps m.
(intermediate head)

Brachial m.

Anconeal m.

Supinator m.

Long abductor of
pollex m.

Deep digital
flexor m.

Long extensor of
pollex m.

Heart

Lungs

Liver

Stomach

Spleen

Interosseous
ligament

Long flexor of
hallux m.

Small intestine
(jejunum)

Capsular m.

Medial vast m.

Femoral adductor m.

PLATE 2.8 Left lateral view deep muscles and in situ viscera of the female.

41

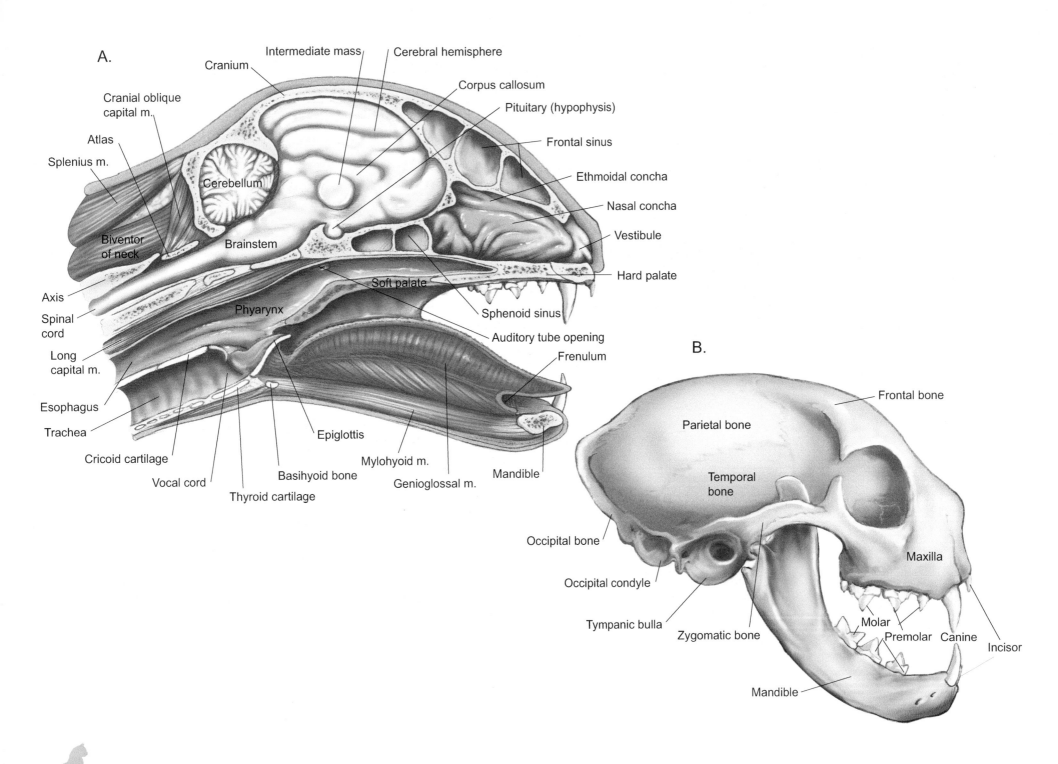

A.

Intermediate mass

Cerebral hemisphere

Cranium

Corpus callosum

Cranial oblique capital m.

Pituitary (hypophysis)

Atlas

Frontal sinus

Splenius m.

Cerebellum

Ethmoidal concha

Nasal concha

Biventor of neck

Brainstem

Vestibule

Axis

Hard palate

Spinal cord

Soft palate

Phyarynx

Sphenoid sinus

Long capital m.

Auditory tube opening

Frenulum

Esophagus

Trachea

Epiglottis

Mylohyoid m.

Cricoid cartilage

Basihyoid bone

Genioglossal m.

Mandible

Vocal cord

Thyroid cartilage

B.

Frontal bone

Parietal bone

Temporal bone

Maxilla

Occipital bone

Occipital condyle

Tympanic bulla

Zygomatic bone

Molar

Premolar

Canine

Incisor

Mandible

PLATE 2.9 A. Median section of the head. B. Skull and dentition

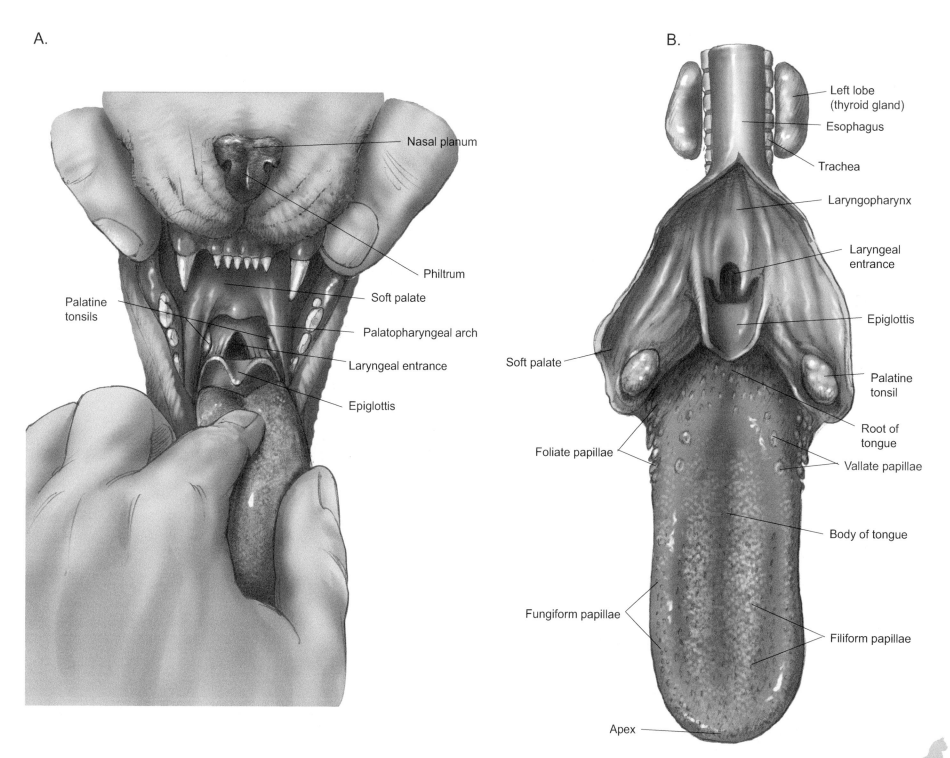

A.

Nasal planum

Philtrum

Soft palate

Palatine
tonsils

Palatopharyngeal arch

Laryngeal entrance

Epiglottis

B.

Left lobe
(thyroid gland)

Esophagus

Trachea

Laryngopharynx

Laryngeal
entrance

Epiglottis

Soft palate

Palatine
tonsil

Root of
tongue

Foliate papillae

Vallate papillae

Body of tongue

Fungiform papillae

Filiform papillae

Apex

PLATE 2.10 Oral cavity: A. View (in situ) of pharynx, tonsils, and epiglottis, B. View (in vivo) tongue, tonsils, pharynx, and epiglottis.

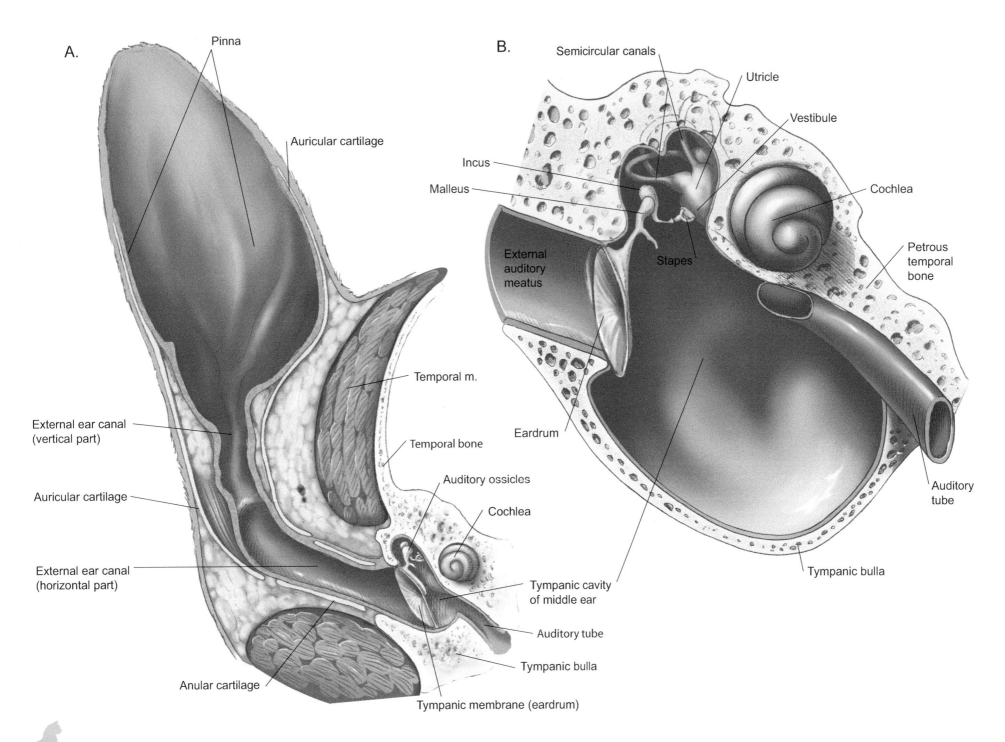

A.

Pinna

Auricular cartilage

Temporal m.

External ear canal
(vertical part)

Temporal bone

Auricular cartilage

Auditory ossicles

Cochlea

External ear canal
(horizontal part)

Tympanic cavity
of middle ear

Auditory tube

Anular cartilage

Tympanic bulla

Tympanic membrane (eardrum)

B.

Semicircular canals

Utricle

Vestibule

Incus

Malleus

Cochlea

External
auditory
meatus

Stapes

Petrous
temporal
bone

Eardrum

Auditory
tube

Tympanic bulla

44 PLATE 2.11 Cat ear: A. The external, middle, and inner ear, B. Middle and inner ear.

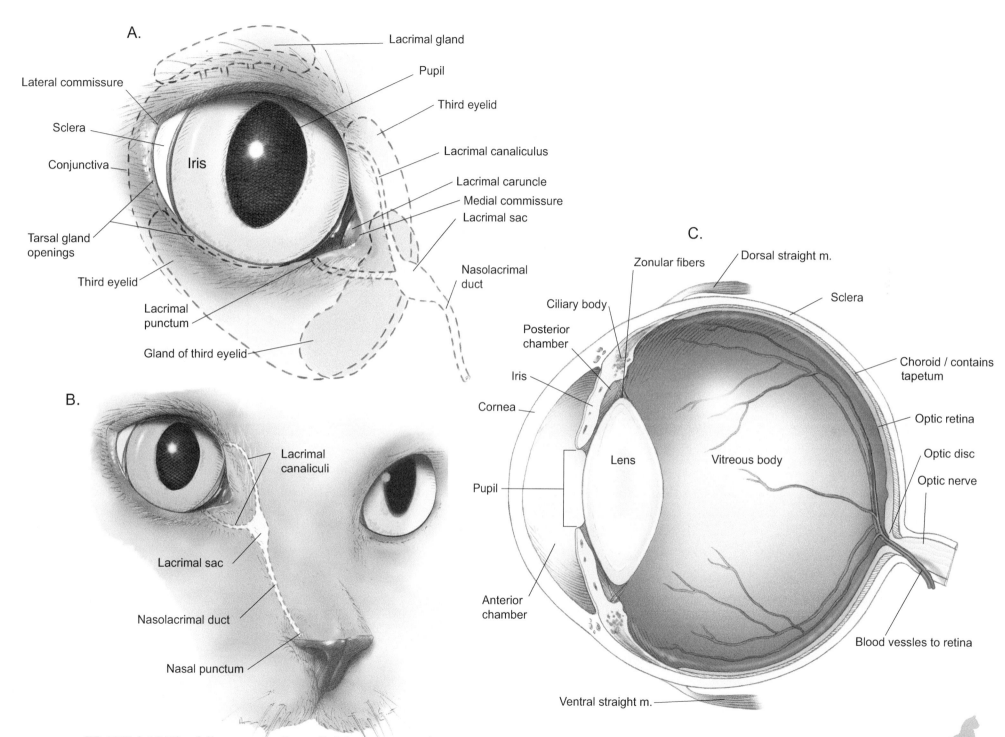

A.

Lacrimal gland

Lateral commissure

Pupil

Third eyelid

Sclera

Lacrimal canaliculus

Iris

Conjunctiva

Lacrimal caruncle

Medial commissure

Lacrimal sac

Tarsal gland openings

Nasolacrimal duct

Third eyelid

Lacrimal punctum

Gland of third eyelid

B.

Lacrimal canaliculi

Lacrimal sac

Nasolacrimal duct

Nasal punctum

C.

Zonular fibers

Dorsal straight m.

Ciliary body

Sclera

Posterior chamber

Iris

Choroid / contains tapetum

Cornea

Optic retina

Pupil

Lens

Vitreous body

Optic disc

Optic nerve

Anterior chamber

Blood vessels to retina

Ventral straight m.

PLATE 2.12 The feline eye: A. Superficial anatomy and accessory structures, B. Nasolacramal apparatus, C. Sagittal section of eyeball.

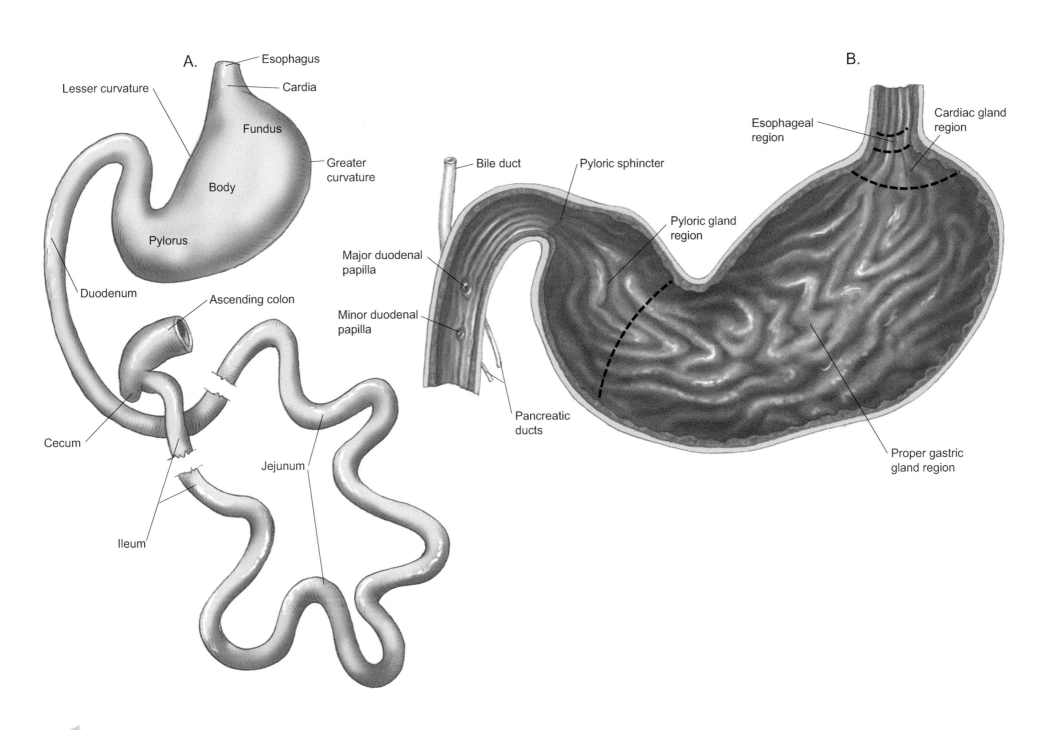

A.

Esophagus

Cardia

Lesser curvature

Fundus

Greater curvature

Body

Pylorus

Duodenum

Ascending colon

Cecum

Jejunum

Ileum

Bile duct

Pyloric sphincter

Major duodenal papilla

Minor duodenal papilla

Pancreatic ducts

B.

Esophageal region

Cardiac gland region

Pyloric gland region

Proper gastric gland region

PLATE 2.13 A. Isolated stomach and intestines. B. Sagittal section of stomach and portion of duodenum.

46

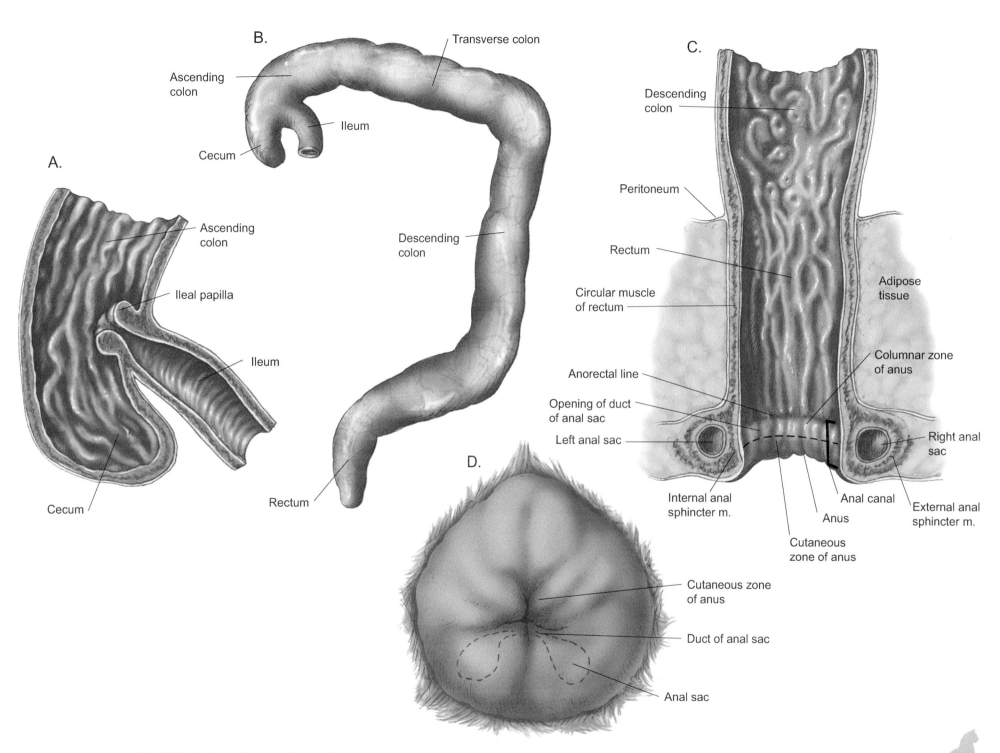

PLATE 2.14 A. Ileocecal junction. B. Gross view of colon. C. Dorsal section of rectum and anus. D. External view of anus.

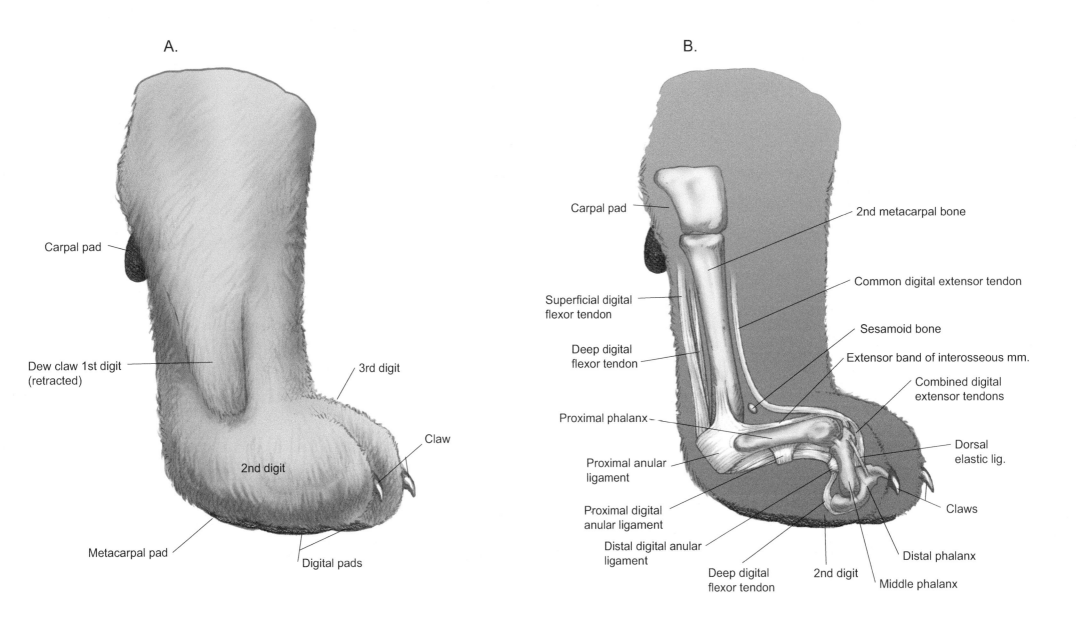

A.

Carpal pad

Dew claw 1st digit
(retracted)

3rd digit

Claw

2nd digit

Metacarpal pad

Digital pads

B.

Carpal pad

2nd metacarpal bone

Common digital extensor tendon

Superficial digital
flexor tendon

Sesamoid bone

Extensor band of interosseous mm.

Deep digital
flexor tendon

Combined digital
extensor tendons

Proximal phalanx

Dorsal
elastic lig.

Proximal anular
ligament

Proximal digital
anular ligament

Claws

Distal digital anular
ligament

Distal phalanx

Deep digital
flexor tendon

2nd digit

Middle phalanx

PLATE 2.15 Forepaw: A. Medial superficial view. B. Medial deep view.

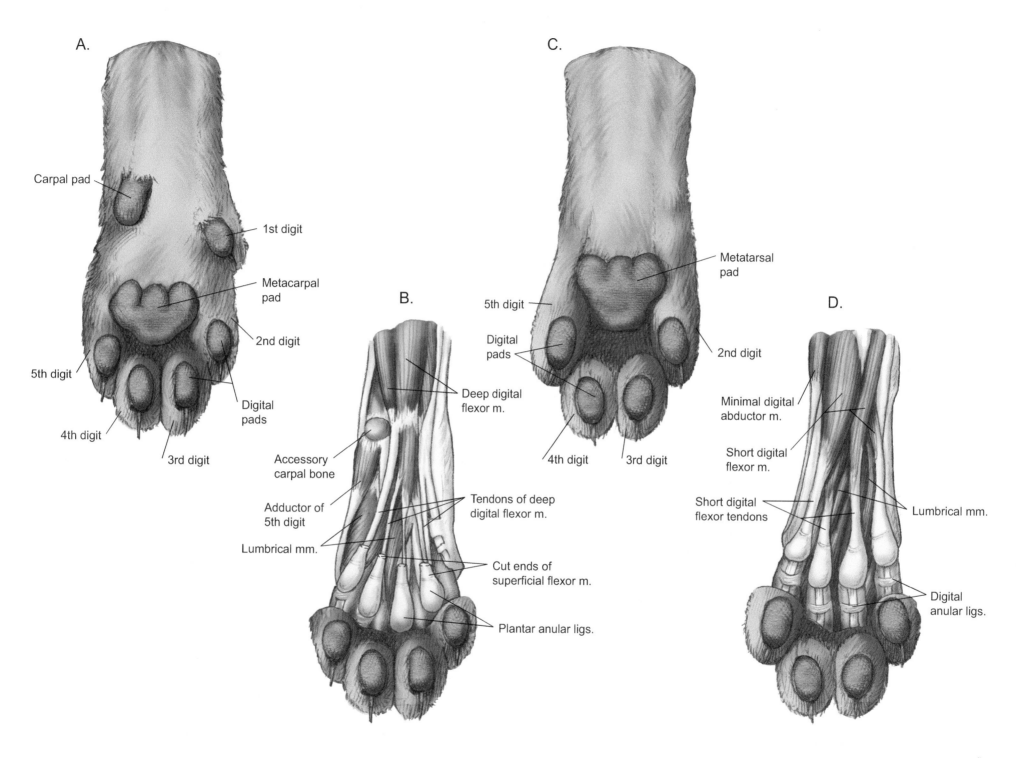

A.

Carpal pad

1st digit

Metacarpal
pad

2nd digit

5th digit

Digital
pads

4th digit

3rd digit

B.

Deep digital
flexor m.

Accessory
carpal bone

Adductor of
5th digit

Lumbrical mm.

Tendons of deep
digital flexor m.

Cut ends of
superficial flexor m.

Plantar anular ligs.

C.

Metatarsal
pad

5th digit

Digital
pads

2nd digit

4th digit

3rd digit

D.

Minimal digital
abductor m.

Short digital
flexor m.

Short digital
flexor tendons

Lumbrical mm.

Digital
anular ligs.

PLATE 2.16 Cat paw: A. Palmar view forepaw, B. Palmar view of deep dissection of forepaw,
C. Plantar view of hindpaw, D. Plantar view of superficial dissection of hindpaw.

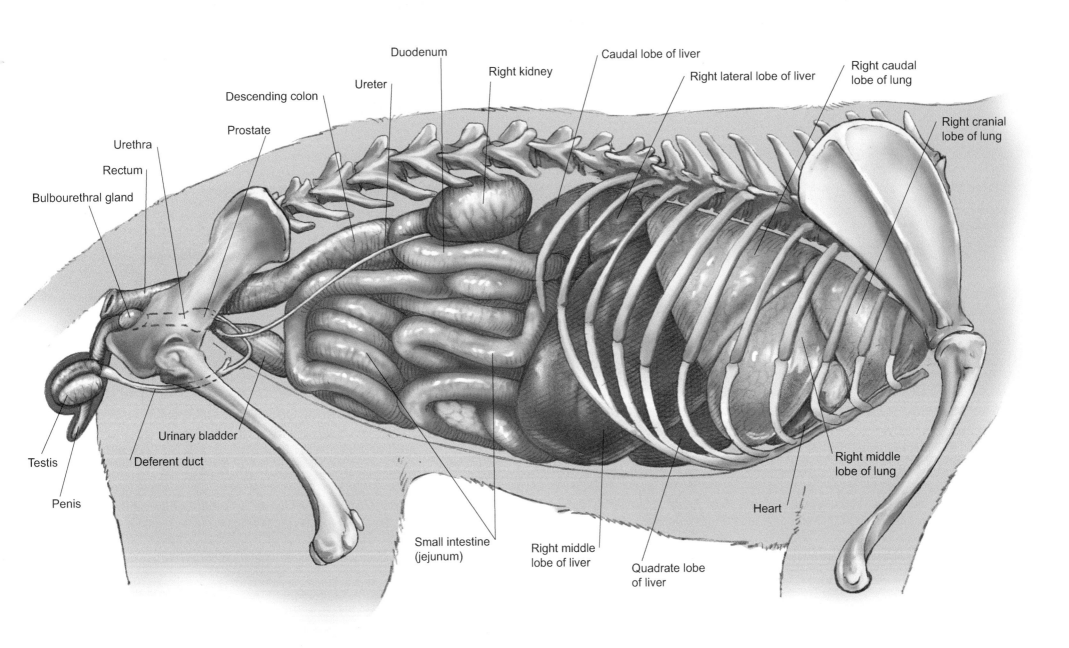

Duodenum

Caudal lobe of liver

Right kidney

Right lateral lobe of liver

Right caudal lobe of lung

Descending colon

Ureter

Right cranial lobe of lung

Prostate

Urethra

Rectum

Bulbourethral gland

Testis

Penis

Urinary bladder

Deferent duct

Small intestine (jejunum)

Right middle lobe of liver

Quadrate lobe of liver

Right middle lobe of lung

Heart

PLATE 2.17 Right lateral view of thoracic, abdominal, and pelvic viscera related to the skeleton of the male.

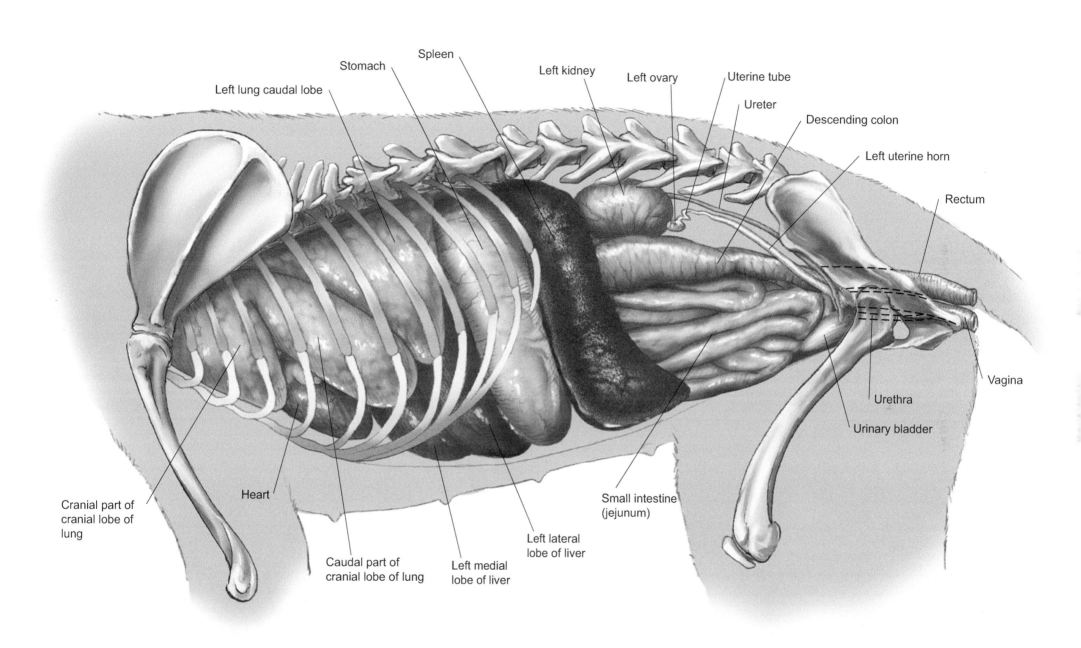

Stomach

Spleen

Left lung caudal lobe

Left kidney

Left ovary

Uterine tube

Ureter

Descending colon

Left uterine horn

Rectum

Cranial part of cranial lobe of lung

Heart

Caudal part of cranial lobe of lung

Left medial lobe of liver

Left lateral lobe of liver

Small intestine (jejunum)

Urethra

Urinary bladder

Vagina

PLATE 2.18 Left lateral view of thoracic, abdominal and pelvic viscera related to the skeleton of the female.

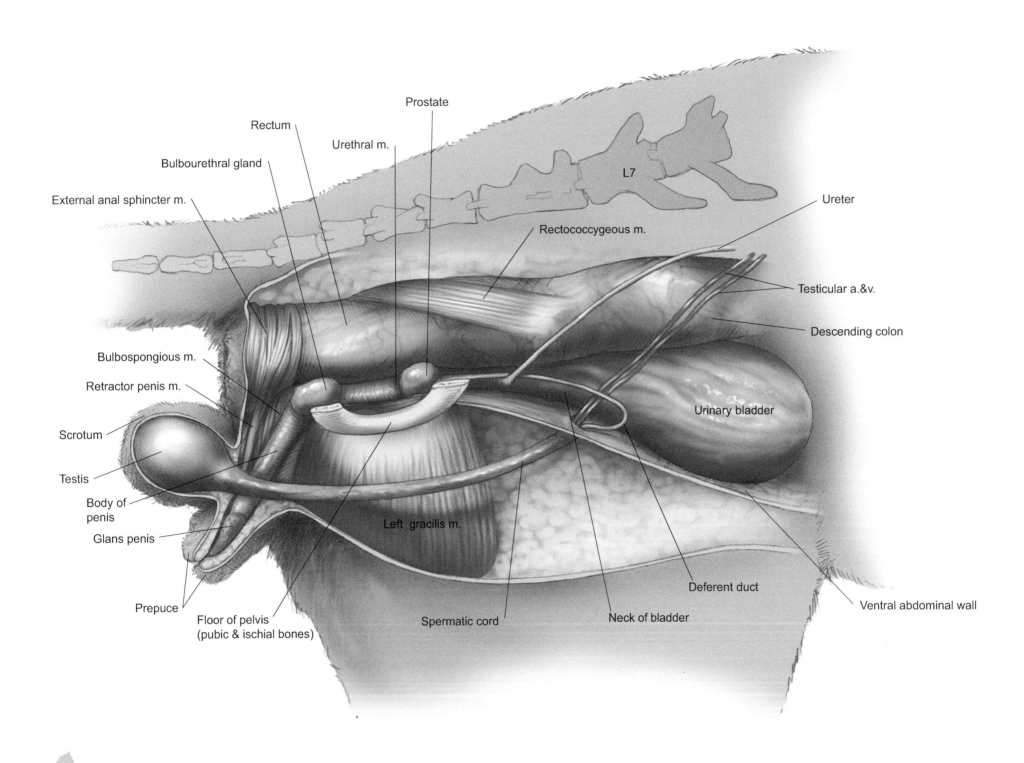

Prostate

Rectum

Urethral m.

Bulbourethral gland

External anal sphincter m.

L7

Ureter

Rectococcygeous m.

Testicular a.&v.

Descending colon

Bulbospongious m.

Retractor penis m.

Scrotum

Urinary bladder

Testis

Body of penis

Glans penis

Left gracilis m.

Prepuce

Deferent duct

Floor of pelvis
(pubic & ischial bones)

Spermatic cord

Neck of bladder

Ventral abdominal wall

PLATE 2.19 Relations of the reproductive organs of the male.

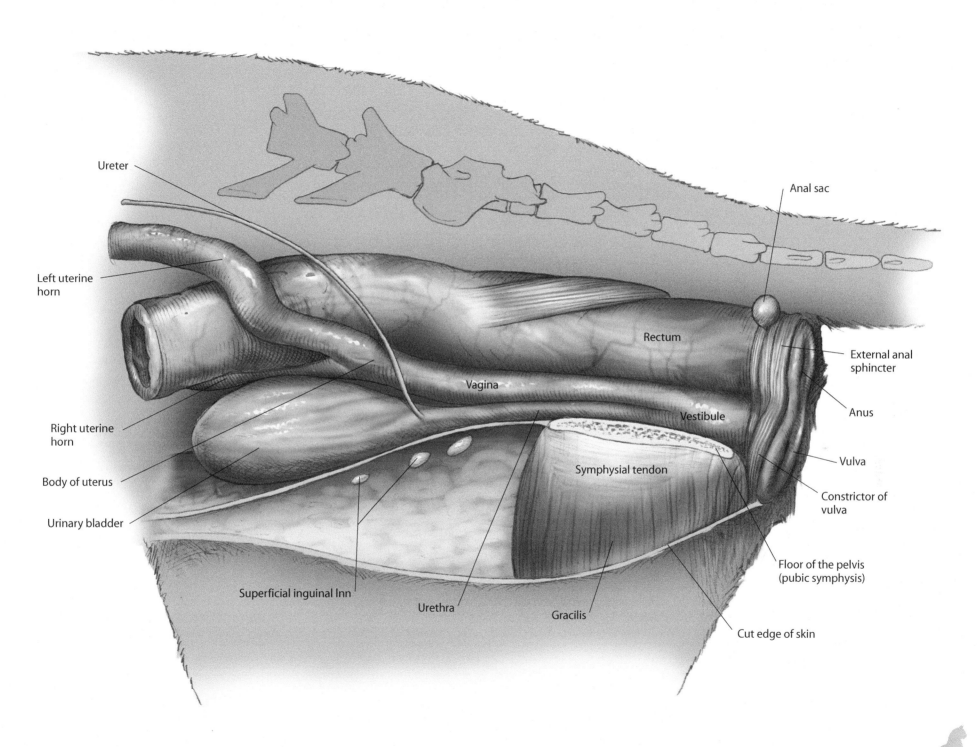

Ureter

Left uterine horn

Right uterine horn

Body of uterus

Urinary bladder

Superficial inguinal lnn

Urethra

Gracilis

Symphysial tendon

Vagina

Rectum

Vestibule

Anal sac

External anal sphincter

Anus

Vulva

Constrictor of vulva

Floor of the pelvis (pubic symphysis)

Cut edge of skin

PLATE 2.20 Left lateral view of the relations of the reproductve organs of the female.

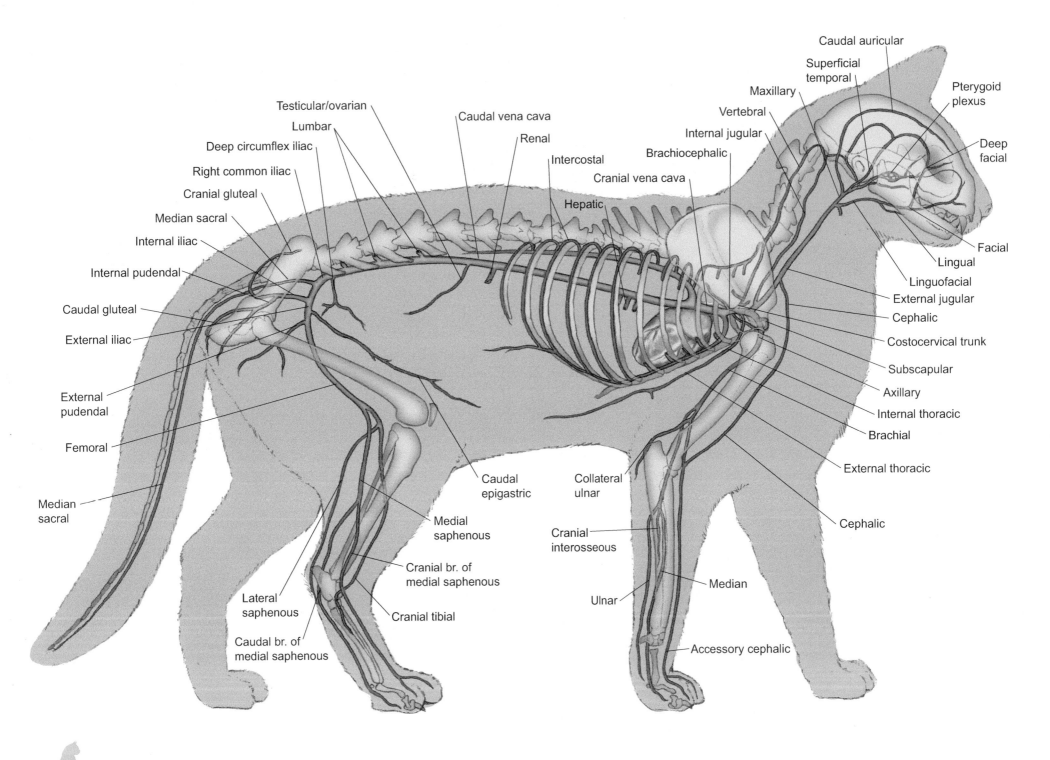

PLATE 2.21 Major veins.

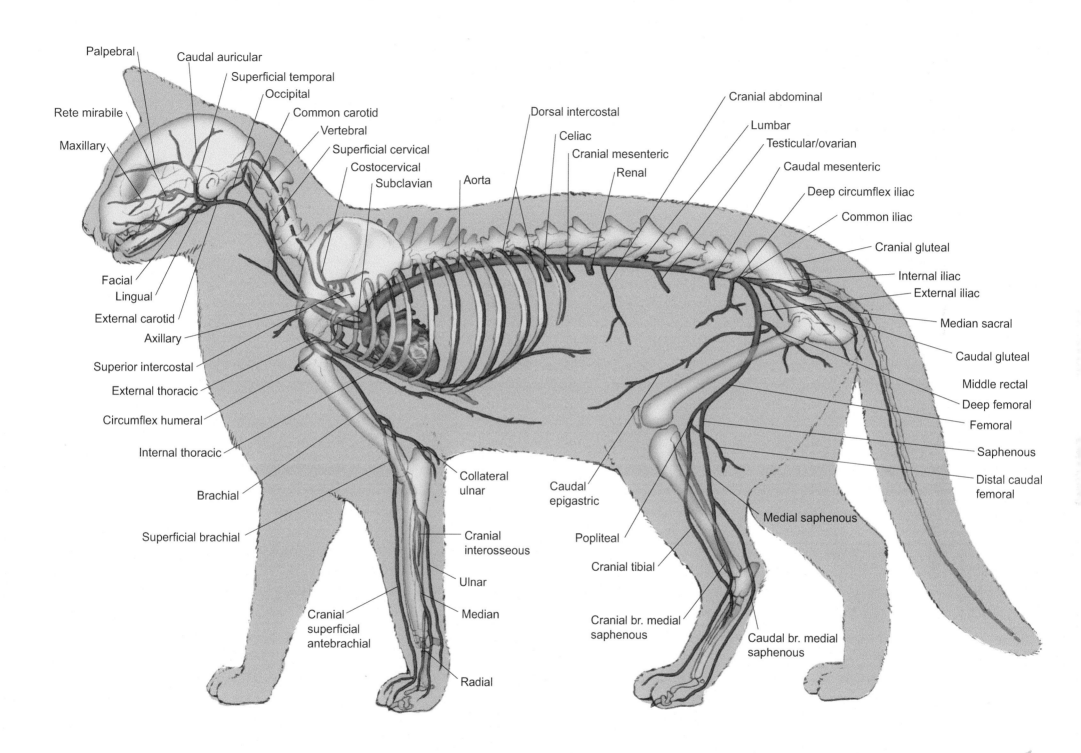

PLATE 2.22 Major arteries.

55

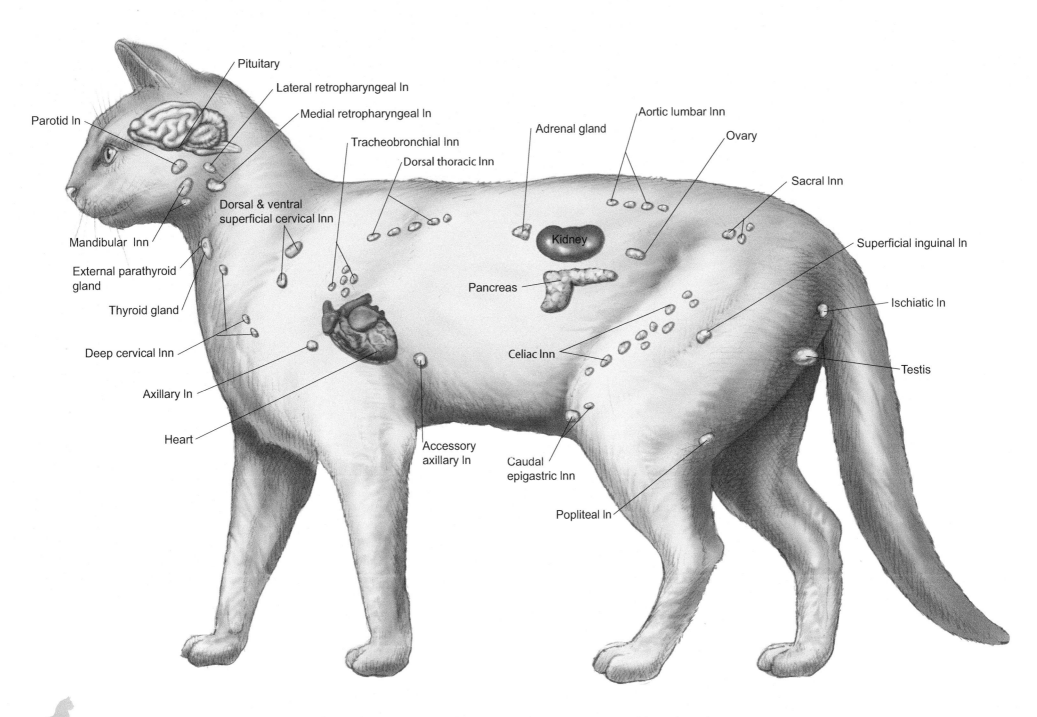

Pituitary

Lateral retropharyngeal ln

Medial retropharyngeal ln

Parotid ln

Aortic lumbar lnn

Adrenal gland

Ovary

Tracheobronchial lnn

Dorsal thoracic lnn

Sacral lnn

Dorsal & ventral
superficial cervical lnn

Mandibular lnn

External parathyroid
gland

Kidney

Superficial inguinal ln

Pancreas

Thyroid gland

Ischiatic ln

Deep cervical lnn

Celiac lnn

Testis

Axillary ln

Heart

Accessory
axillary ln

Caudal
epigastric lnn

Popliteal ln

56

PLATE 2.23 Endocrine organs and peripheral lymph nodes.

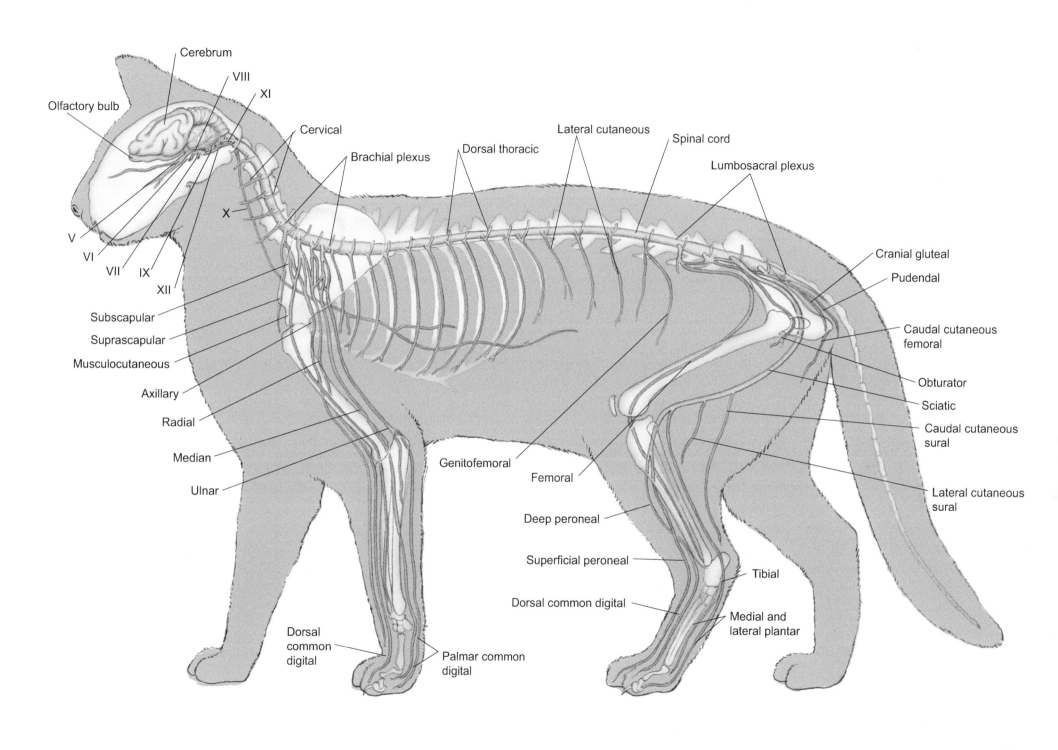

Plate 2.24 Central and peripheral nervous systems. I-olfactory, II-optic, III-oculomotor, IV-trochlear, V-trigeminal, VI-abducens, VII-facial, VIII-vestibulocochlear, IX-glossopharyngeal, X-vagus, XI-hypoglossal, XII-accessory nerves.

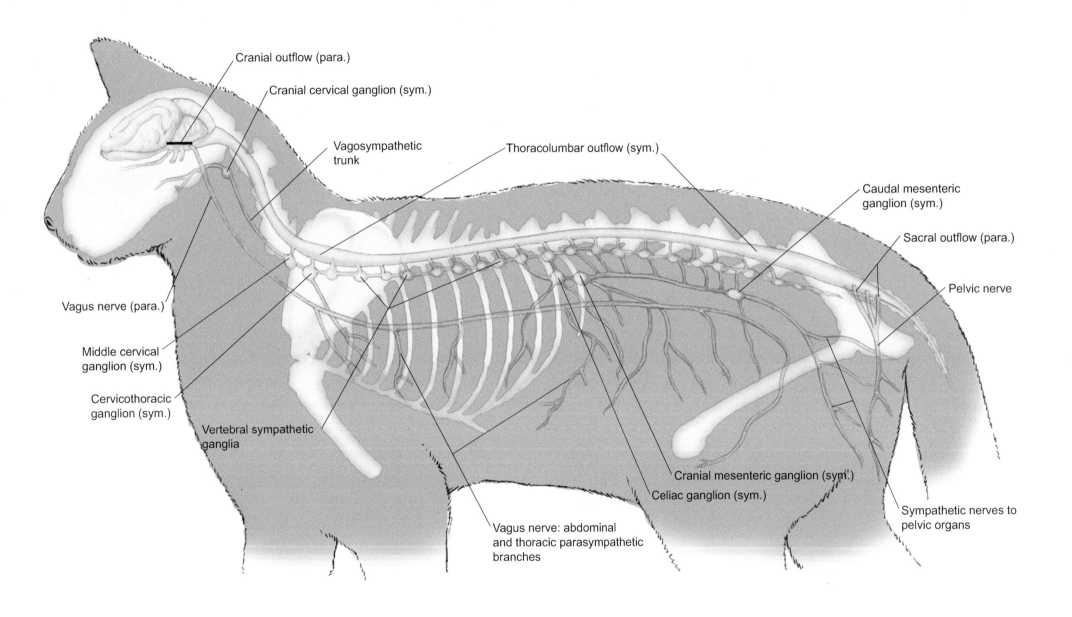

Cranial outflow (para.)

Cranial cervical ganglion (sym.)

Vagosympathetic trunk

Thoracolumbar outflow (sym.)

Caudal mesenteric ganglion (sym.)

Sacral outflow (para.)

Vagus nerve (para.)

Pelvic nerve

Middle cervical ganglion (sym.)

Cervicothoracic ganglion (sym.)

Vertebral sympathetic ganglia

Cranial mesenteric ganglion (sym.)

Celiac ganglion (sym.)

Vagus nerve: abdominal and thoracic parasympathetic branches

Sympathetic nerves to pelvic organs

Plate 2.25 Autonomic nervous system: Sym. = sympathetic division and Para. = parasympathetic division.

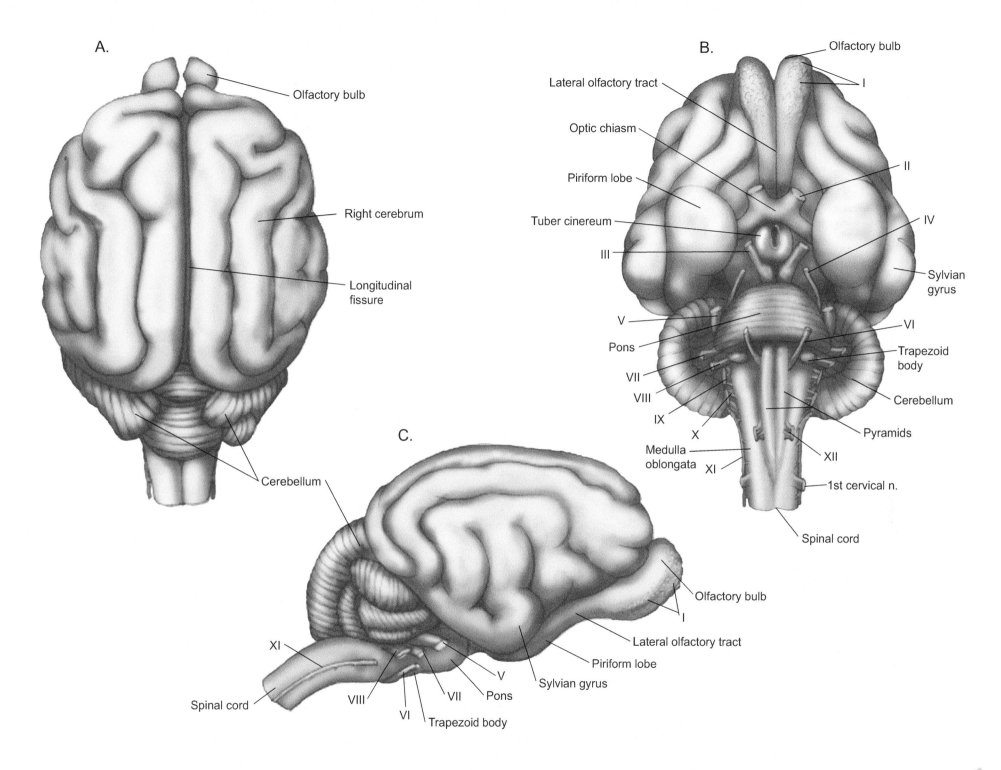

A.

Olfactory bulb

Right cerebrum

Longitudinal fissure

Cerebellum

B.

Olfactory bulb

Lateral olfactory tract

I

Optic chiasm

II

Piriform lobe

Tuber cinereum

III

IV

Sylvian gyrus

V

Pons

VI

Trapezoid body

VII

VIII

IX

Cerebellum

X

Pyramids

Medulla oblongata

XI

XII

1st cervical n.

Spinal cord

C.

XI

Spinal cord

VIII

VI

Trapezoid body

V

VII

Pons

Sylvian gyrus

Piriform lobe

Lateral olfactory tract

Olfactory bulb

I

Plate 2.26 Brain: A. Dorsal view, B. Ventral view, C. Lateral view. I-olfactory, II-optic, III-oculomotor, IV-trochlear, V-trigeminal, VI-abducens, VII-facial, VIII-vestibulocochlear, IX-glossopharyngeal, X-vagus, XI-accessory, XII-hypoglossal nerves.

SECTION 3   THE RABBIT

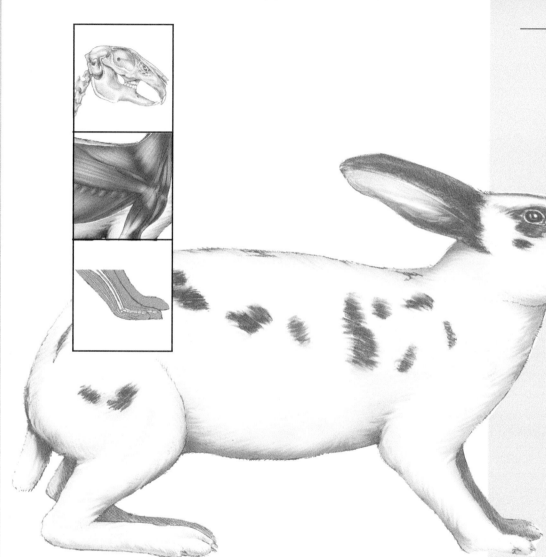

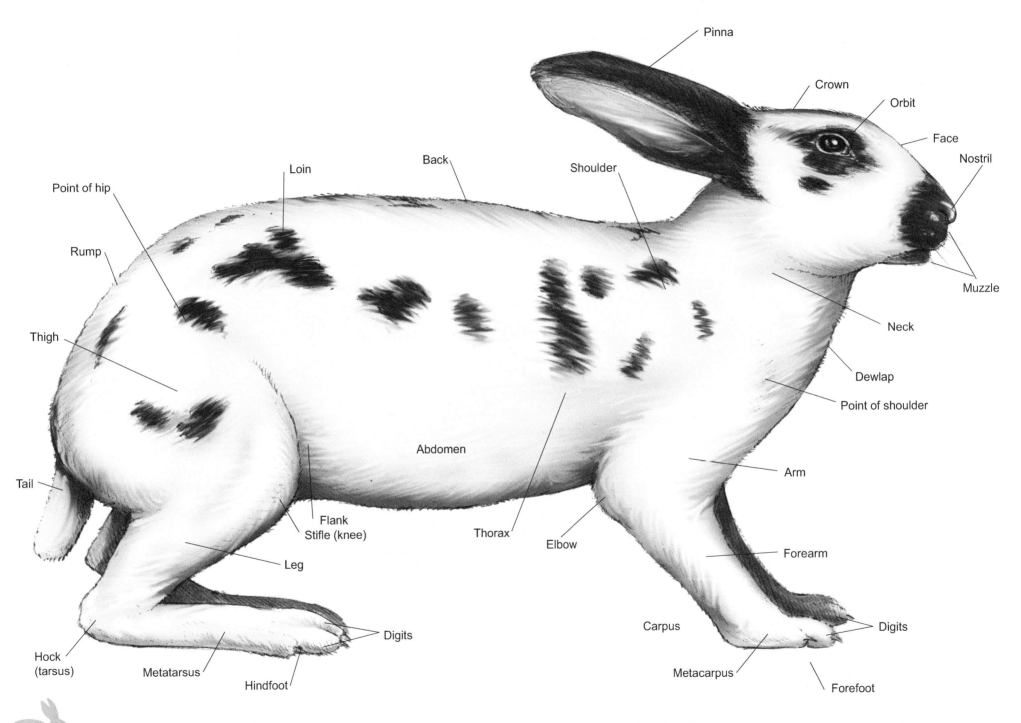

Plate 3.1 Lateral view of the male rabbit (Dalmatian Rex).

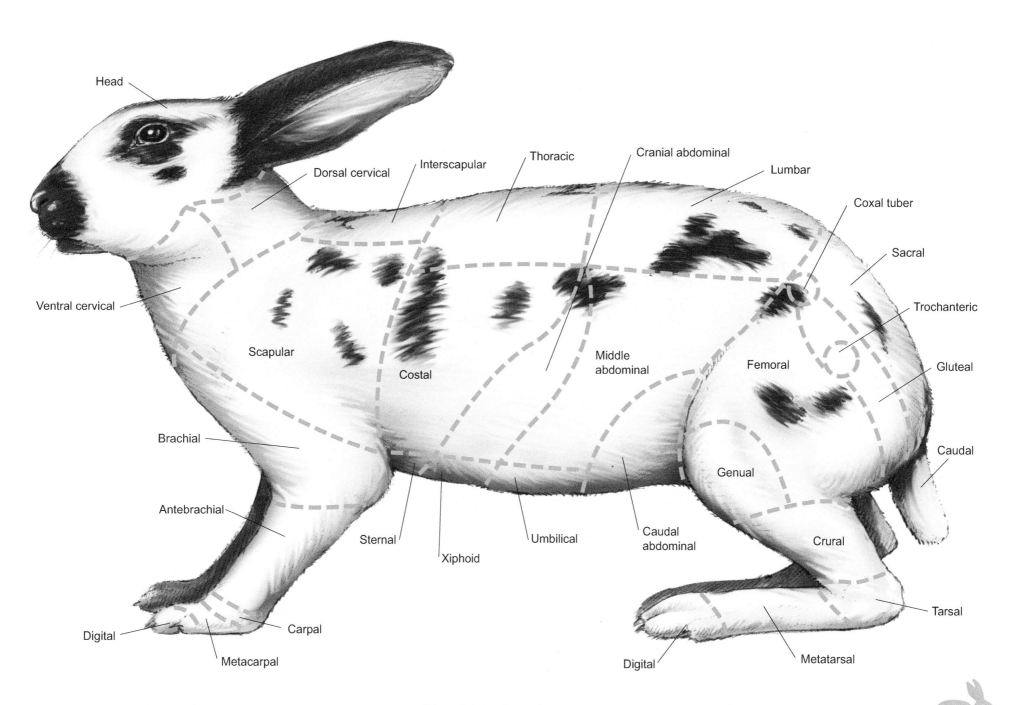

Plate 3.2 Body regions.

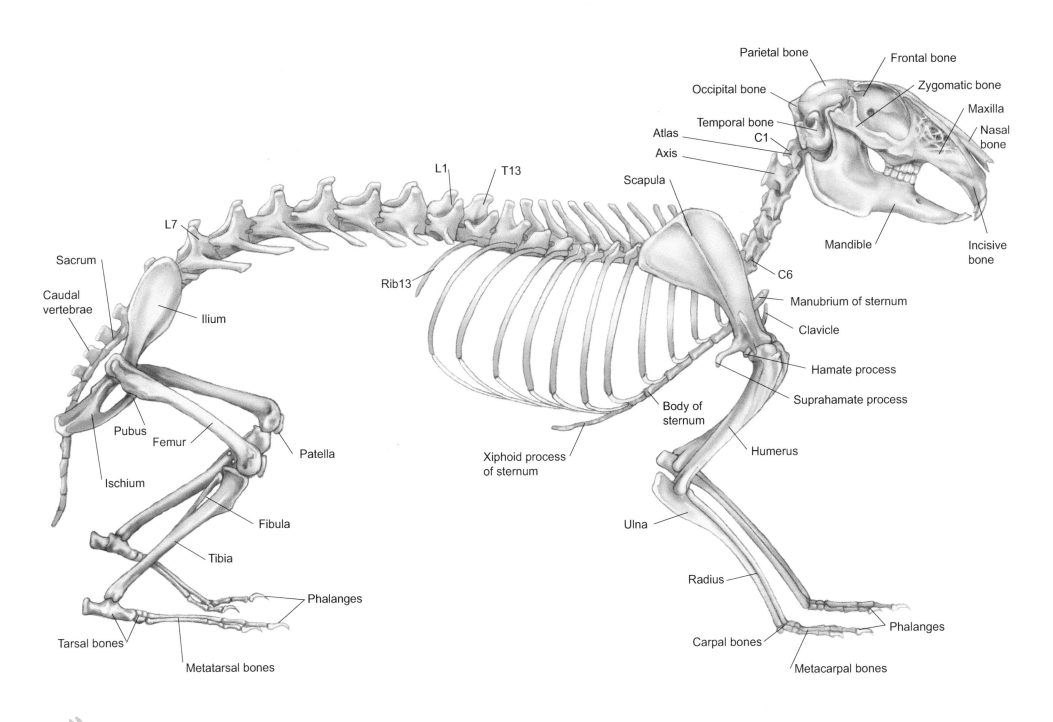

Parietal bone

Frontal bone

Occipital bone

Zygomatic bone

Maxilla

Temporal bone

Nasal bone

Atlas

C1

Axis

Scapula

Mandible

Incisive bone

L1

T13

L7

C6

Sacrum

Rib13

Manubrium of sternum

Caudal vertebrae

Clavicle

Ilium

Hamate process

Pubus

Suprahamate process

Ischium

Femur

Patella

Body of sternum

Humerus

Fibula

Xiphoid process of sternum

Tibia

Ulna

Phalanges

Radius

Phalanges

Tarsal bones

Carpal bones

Metatarsal bones

Metacarpal bones

Plate 3.3 Skeleton; C = Cervical vertebrae, T = Thoracic vertebrae, L = Lumbar vertebrae.

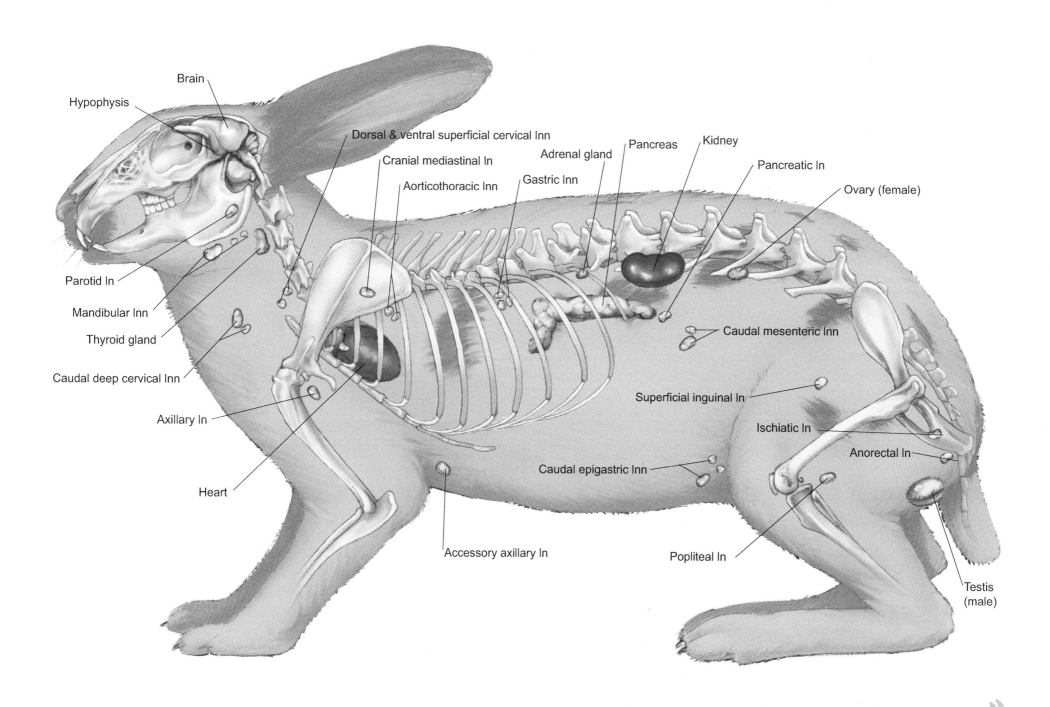

Plate 3.4 Endocrine organs and lymph nodes.

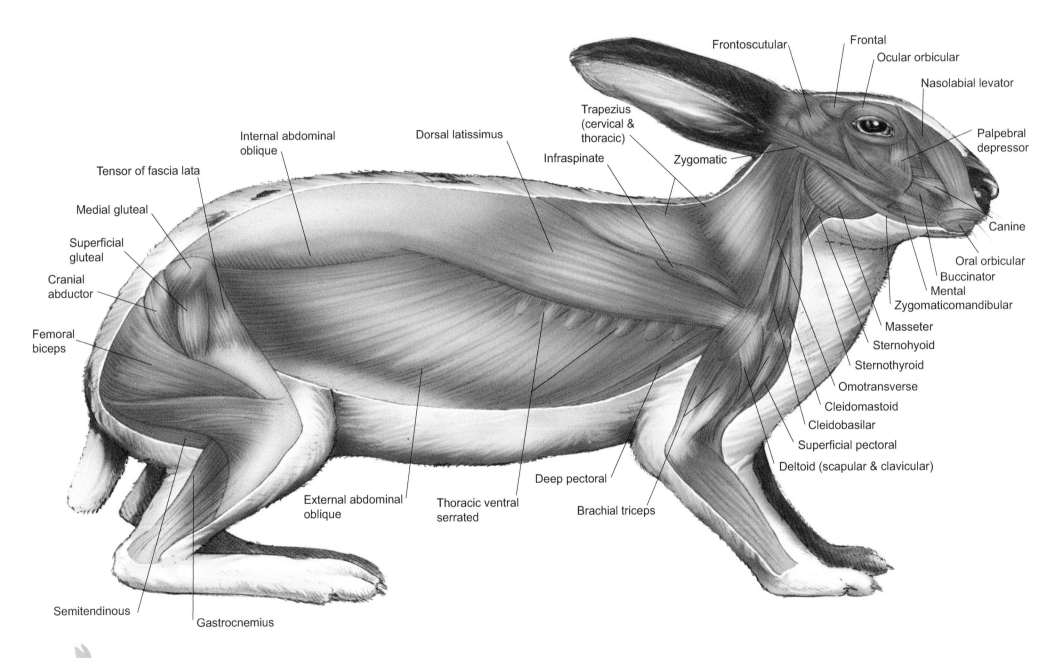

Frontoscutular

Frontal

Ocular orbicular

Nasolabial levator

Trapezius (cervical & thoracic)

Palpebral depressor

Infraspinate

Zygomatic

Internal abdominal oblique

Dorsal latissimus

Tensor of fascia lata

Canine

Medial gluteal

Oral orbicular

Superficial gluteal

Buccinator

Cranial abductor

Mental

Zygomaticomandibular

Masseter

Femoral biceps

Sternohyoid

Sternothyroid

Omotransverse

Cleidomastoid

Cleidobasilar

Superficial pectoral

Deltoid (scapular & clavicular)

Deep pectoral

Semitendinous

External abdominal oblique

Thoracic ventral serrated

Brachial triceps

Gastrocnemius

Plate 3.5 Superficial muscles of the male.

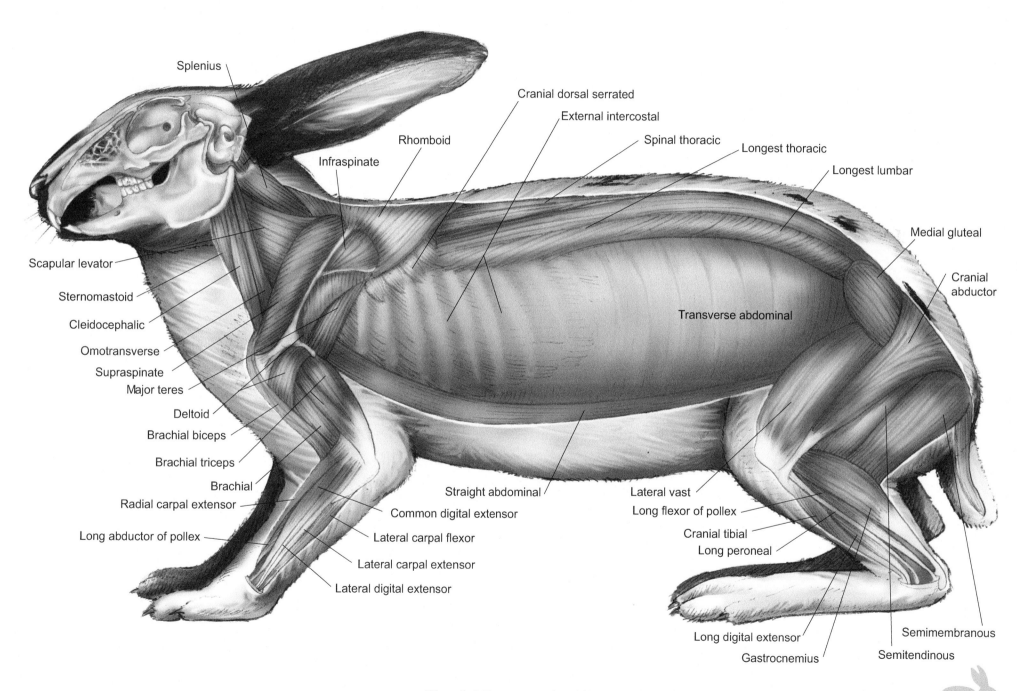

Splenius

Cranial dorsal serrated

External intercostal

Rhomboid

Spinal thoracic

Longest thoracic

Infraspinate

Longest lumbar

Scapular levator

Medial gluteal

Sternomastoid

Cranial
abductor

Cleidocephalic

Omotransverse

Transverse abdominal

Supraspinate

Major teres

Deltoid

Brachial biceps

Brachial triceps

Brachial

Lateral vast

Radial carpal extensor

Straight abdominal

Long flexor of pollex

Long abductor of pollex

Common digital extensor

Cranial tibial

Lateral carpal flexor

Long peroneal

Lateral carpal extensor

Lateral digital extensor

Long digital extensor

Semimembranous

Gastrocnemius

Semitendinous

Plate 3.6 Deep muscles of the female.

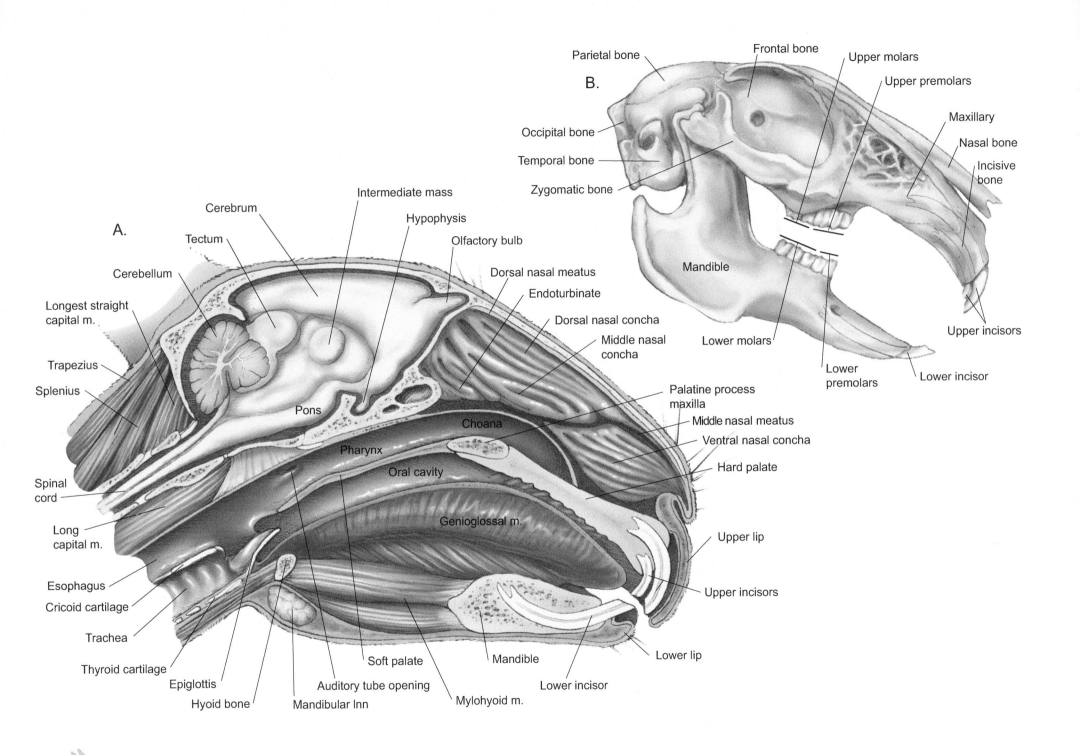

Plate 3.7 A. Median section of the head. B. Skull and dentition.

A.

Cerebrum
Tectum
Cerebellum
Longest straight capital m.
Trapezius
Splenius
Spinal cord
Long capital m.
Esophagus
Cricoid cartilage
Trachea
Thyroid cartilage
Epiglottis
Hyoid bone
Mandibular lnn
Pons

Intermediate mass
Hypophysis
Olfactory bulb
Dorsal nasal meatus
Endoturbinate
Dorsal nasal concha
Middle nasal concha

Pharynx
Oral cavity
Choana
Genioglossal m.

Soft palate
Auditory tube opening
Mylohyoid m.
Mandible
Lower incisor

Palatine process maxilla
Middle nasal meatus
Ventral nasal concha
Hard palate

Upper lip
Upper incisors
Lower lip

B.

Parietal bone
Frontal bone
Upper molars
Upper premolars
Occipital bone
Maxillary
Temporal bone
Nasal bone
Zygomatic bone
Incisive bone

Mandible
Lower molars
Lower premolars
Upper incisors
Lower incisor

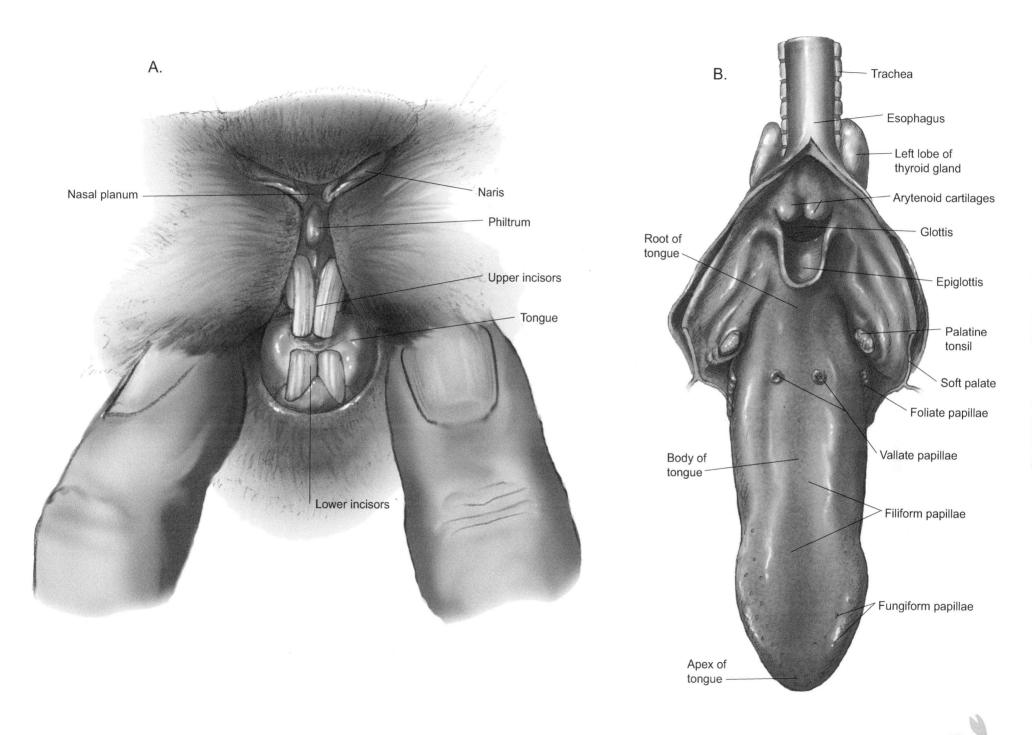

A.

Nasal planum

Naris

Philtrum

Upper incisors

Tongue

Lower incisors

B.

Trachea

Esophagus

Left lobe of
thyroid gland

Arytenoid cartilages

Glottis

Root of
tongue

Epiglottis

Palatine
tonsil

Soft palate

Foliate papillae

Vallate papillae

Body of
tongue

Filiform papillae

Fungiform papillae

Apex of
tongue

Plate 3.8 Oral cavity: A. Teeth and nose, B. Tongue, pharynx, and esophagus.

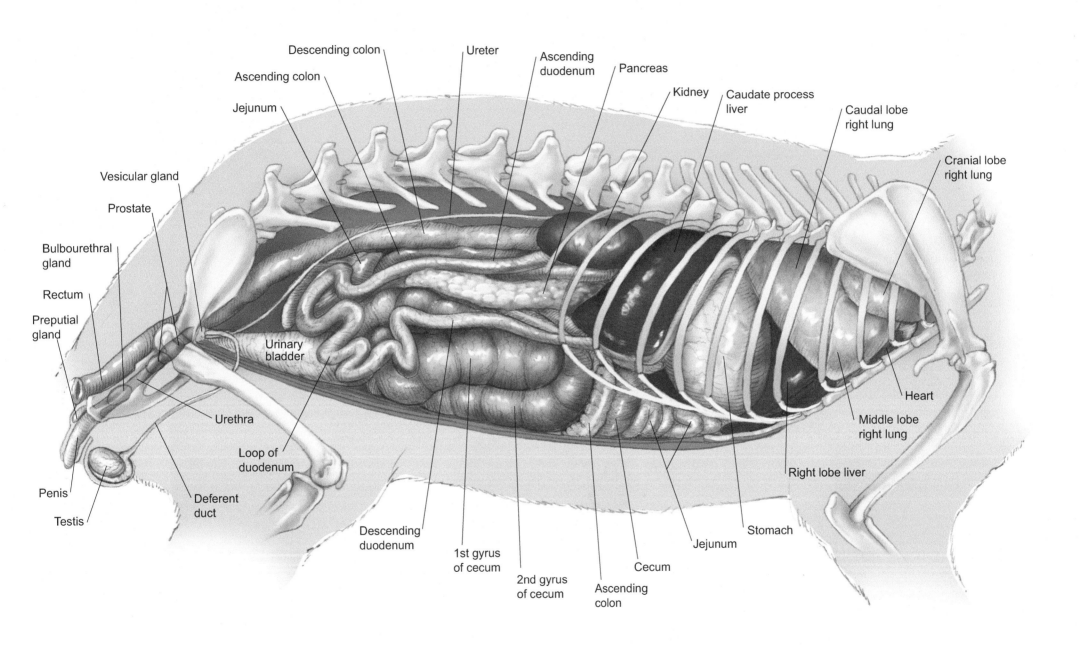

Descending colon

Ascending colon

Jejunum

Vesicular gland

Prostate

Bulbourethral
gland

Rectum

Preputial
gland

Penis

Testis

Urethra

Deferent
duct

Loop of
duodenum

Urinary
bladder

Descending
duodenum

1st gyrus
of cecum

2nd gyrus
of cecum

Ascending
colon

Cecum

Jejunum

Stomach

Ureter

Ascending
duodenum

Pancreas

Kidney

Caudate process
liver

Caudal lobe
right lung

Cranial lobe
right lung

Heart

Middle lobe
right lung

Right lobe liver

70

Plate 3.9 Thoracic, abdominal and pelvic viscera (in situ) of the male. Right lateral view.

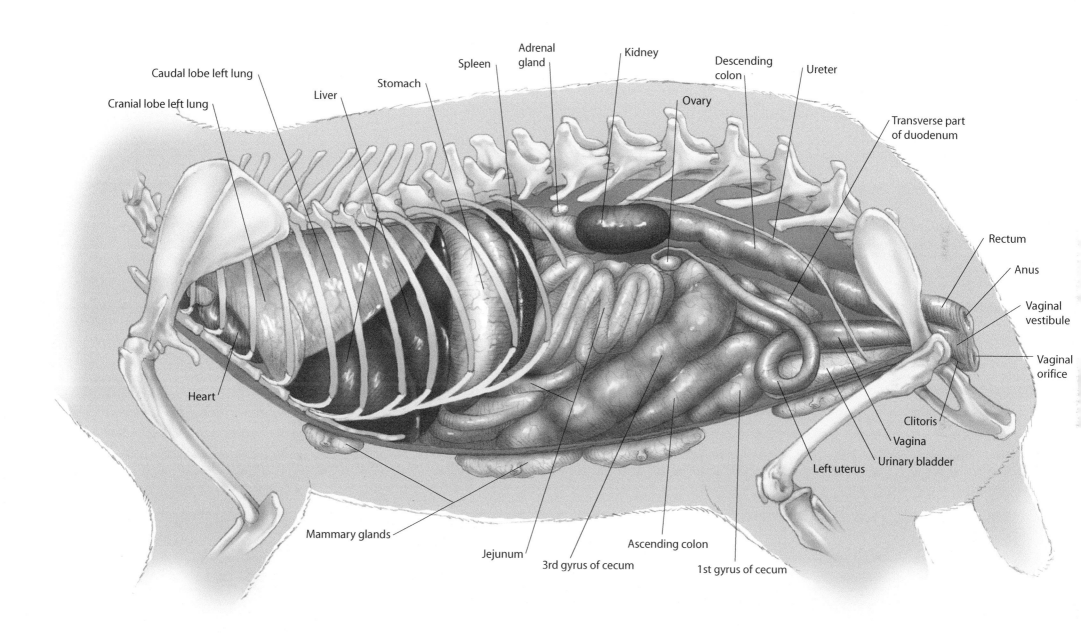

Caudal lobe left lung

Cranial lobe left lung

Liver

Stomach

Spleen

Adrenal gland

Kidney

Ovary

Descending colon

Ureter

Transverse part of duodenum

Rectum

Anus

Vaginal vestibule

Vaginal orifice

Clitoris

Vagina

Urinary bladder

Left uterus

Heart

Mammary glands

Jejunum

3rd gyrus of cecum

Ascending colon

1st gyrus of cecum

Plate 3.10 Thoracic, abdominal, and pelvic viscera (in situ) of the female. Left lateral view.

71

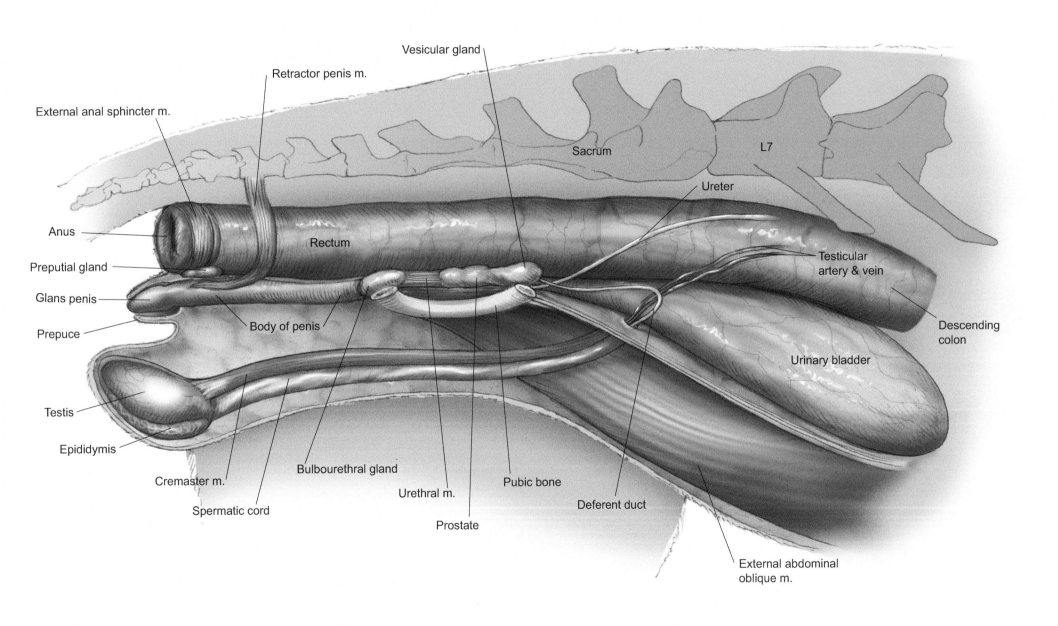

Vesicular gland

Retractor penis m.

External anal sphincter m.

Sacrum

L7

Ureter

Anus

Rectum

Testicular
artery & vein

Preputial gland

Glans penis

Prepuce

Body of penis

Descending
colon

Urinary bladder

Testis

Epididymis

Cremaster m.

Bulbourethral gland

Pubic bone

Spermatic cord

Urethral m.

Deferent duct

Prostate

External abdominal
oblique m.

Plate 3.11 Relations of the reproductive organs of the male.

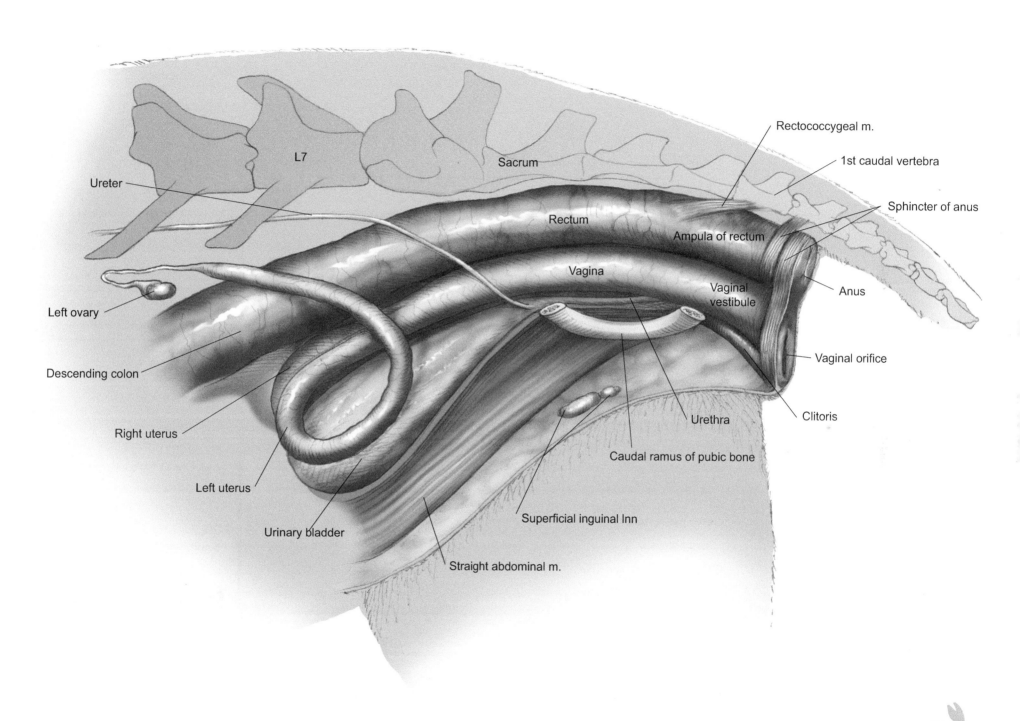

Plate 3.12 Relations of the reproductive organs of the female.

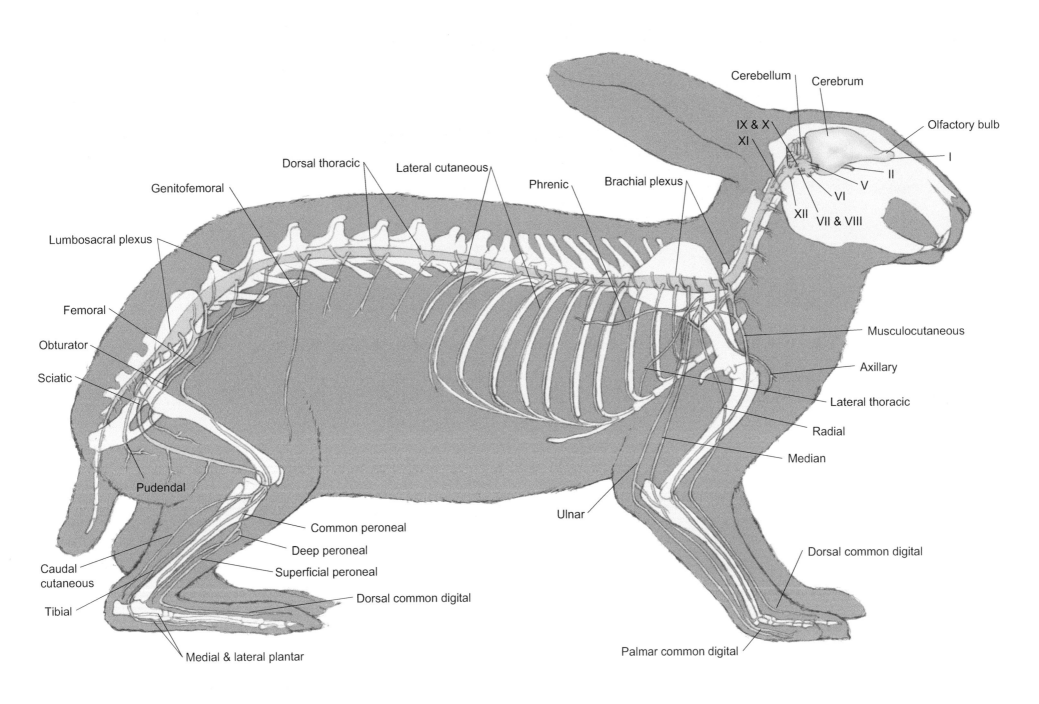

Plate 3.13 Central and peripheral nervous system. I-olfactory, II-optic, III-oculomotor, IV-trochlear, V-trigeminal, VI-abducens, VII-facial, VIII-vestibulocochlear, IX-glossopharyngeal, X-vagus, XI-hypoglossal, XII-accessory nerves.

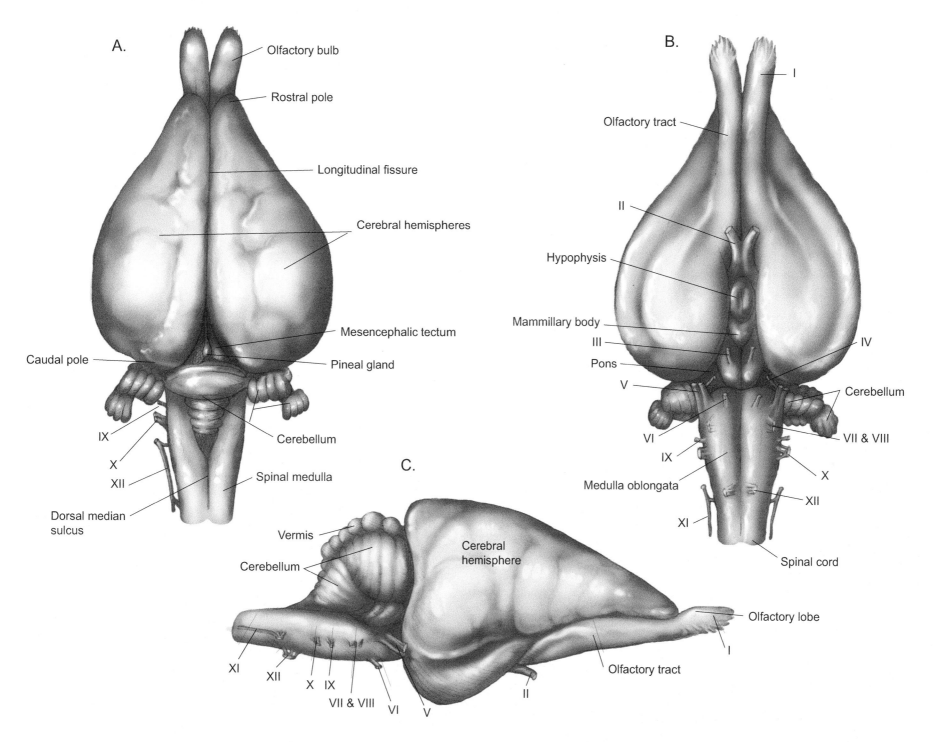

A.

Olfactory bulb

Rostral pole

Longitudinal fissure

Cerebral hemispheres

Mesencephalic tectum

Caudal pole

Pineal gland

IX

X

XII

Cerebellum

Spinal medulla

Dorsal median sulcus

B.

I

Olfactory tract

II

Hypophysis

Mammillary body

III

Pons

V

VI

IX

Medulla oblongata

XI

IV

Cerebellum

VII & VIII

X

XII

Spinal cord

C.

Vermis

Cerebellum

Cerebral hemisphere

Olfactory lobe

XI

XII

X

IX

VII & VIII

VI

V

II

Olfactory tract

I

Plate 3.14 Brain: A. dorsal view, B. ventral view, C. lateral view. I-olfactory, II-optic, III-oculomotor, IV-trochlear, V-trigeminal, VI-abducens, VII-facial, VIII-vestibulocochlear, IX-glossopharyngeal, X-vagus, XI-hypoglossal, XII-accessory nerves.

SECTION 4 THE RAT

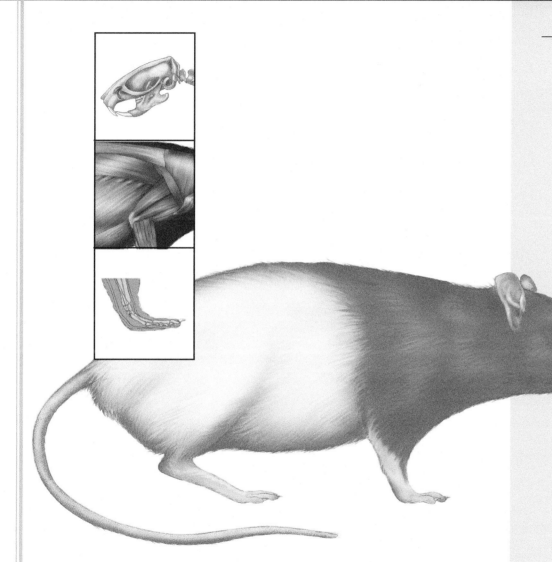

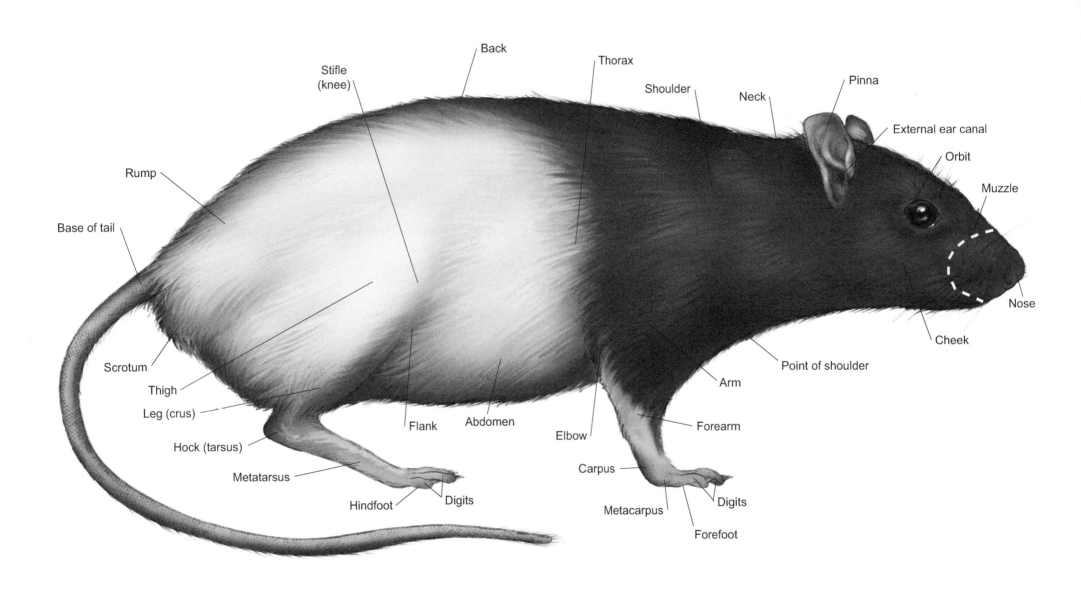

Back

Thorax

Stifle
(knee)

Shoulder

Neck

Pinna

External ear canal

Orbit

Rump

Muzzle

Base of tail

Nose

Cheek

Scrotum

Point of shoulder

Thigh

Arm

Leg (crus)

Forearm

Hock (tarsus)

Flank

Abdomen

Elbow

Metatarsus

Carpus

Digits

Hindfoot

Digits

Metacarpus

Forefoot

Plate 4.1 Lateral view. of male rat (Hooded)

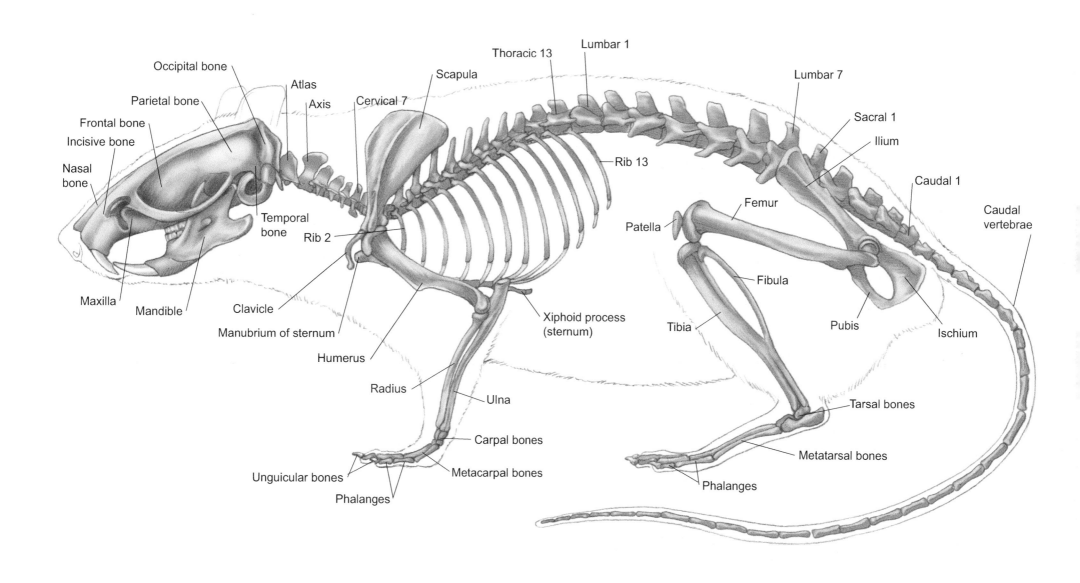

Plate 4.2 Skeleton.

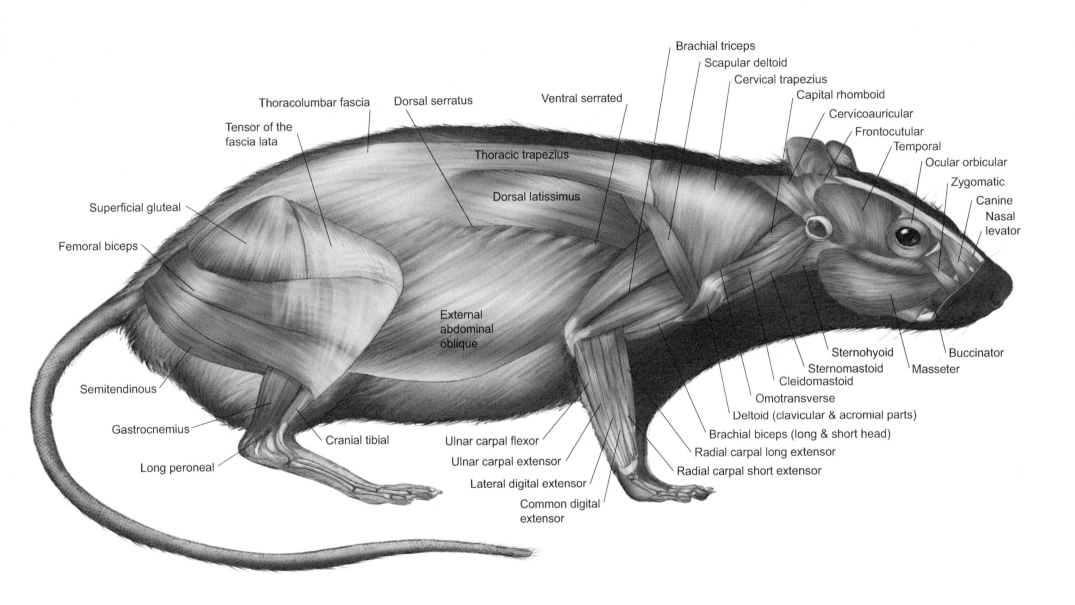

Brachial triceps

Scapular deltoid

Cervical trapezius

Capital rhomboid

Cervicoauricular

Frontocutular

Temporal

Ocular orbicular

Zygomatic

Canine

Nasal
levator

Thoracolumbar fascia

Dorsal serratus

Ventral serrated

Tensor of the
fascia lata

Thoracic trapezius

Dorsal latissimus

Superficial gluteal

Femoral biceps

External
abdominal
oblique

Sternohyoid

Buccinator

Sternomastoid

Masseter

Semitendinous

Cleidomastoid

Gastrocnemius

Omotransverse

Cranial tibial

Deltoid (clavicular & acromial parts)

Ulnar carpal flexor

Brachial biceps (long & short head)

Long peroneal

Ulnar carpal extensor

Radial carpal long extensor

Lateral digital extensor

Radial carpal short extensor

Common digital
extensor

Plate 4.3 Right lateral view of superficial muscles of the male.

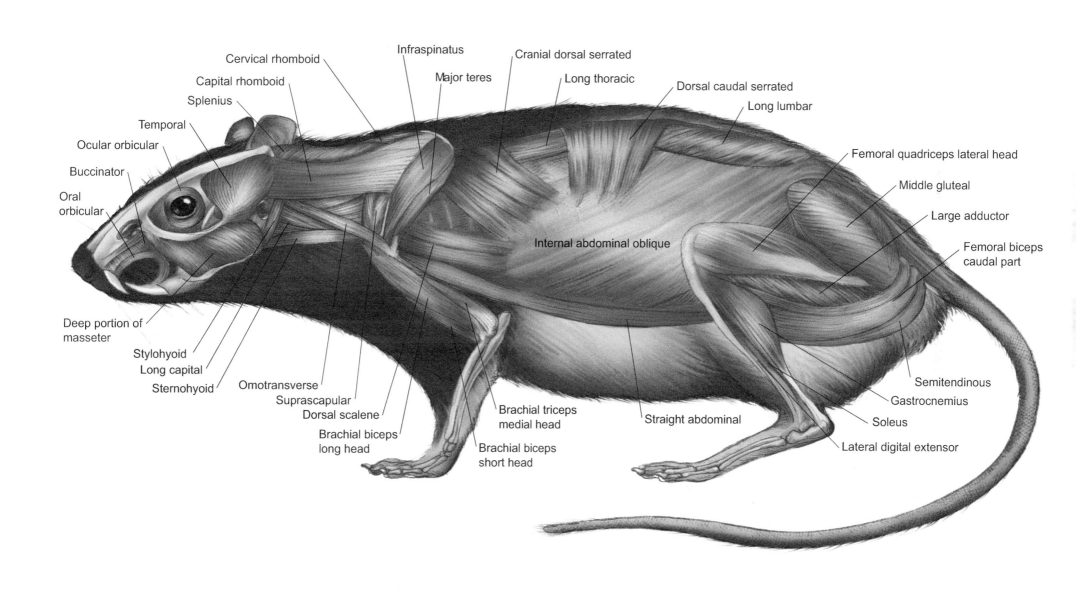

Plate 4.4 Left lateral view of middle and deep muscles of the female.

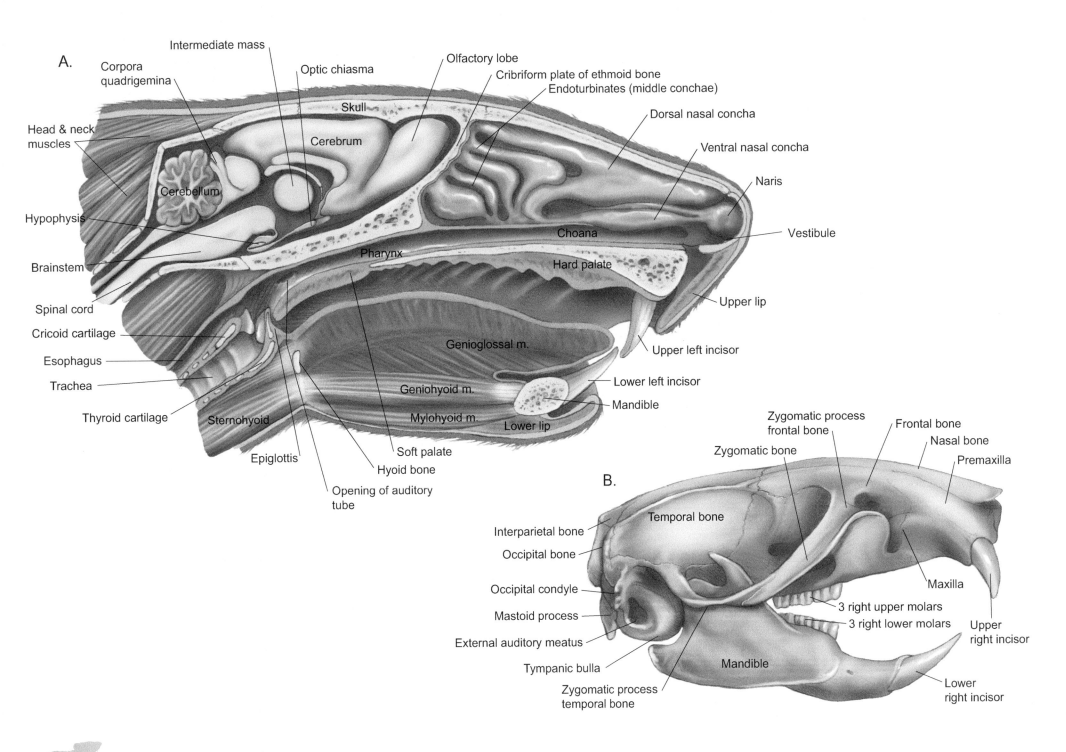

A.

Intermediate mass

Corpora quadrigemina

Optic chiasma

Olfactory lobe

Cribriform plate of ethmoid bone

Endoturbinates (middle conchae)

Skull

Dorsal nasal concha

Head & neck muscles

Cerebrum

Ventral nasal concha

Cerebellum

Naris

Hypophysis

Choana

Vestibule

Brainstem

Pharynx

Hard palate

Spinal cord

Upper lip

Cricoid cartilage

Genioglossal m.

Upper left incisor

Esophagus

Lower left incisor

Trachea

Geniohyoid m.

Mandible

Thyroid cartilage

Sternohyoid

Mylohyoid m.

Lower lip

Epiglottis

Soft palate

Hyoid bone

Opening of auditory tube

B.

Zygomatic process frontal bone

Frontal bone

Nasal bone

Zygomatic bone

Premaxilla

Interparietal bone

Temporal bone

Occipital bone

Occipital condyle

Mastoid process

Maxilla

External auditory meatus

3 right upper molars

3 right lower molars

Tympanic bulla

Mandible

Upper right incisor

Zygomatic process temporal bone

Lower right incisor

Plate 4.5 A. Median section of head. B. Skull and teeth.

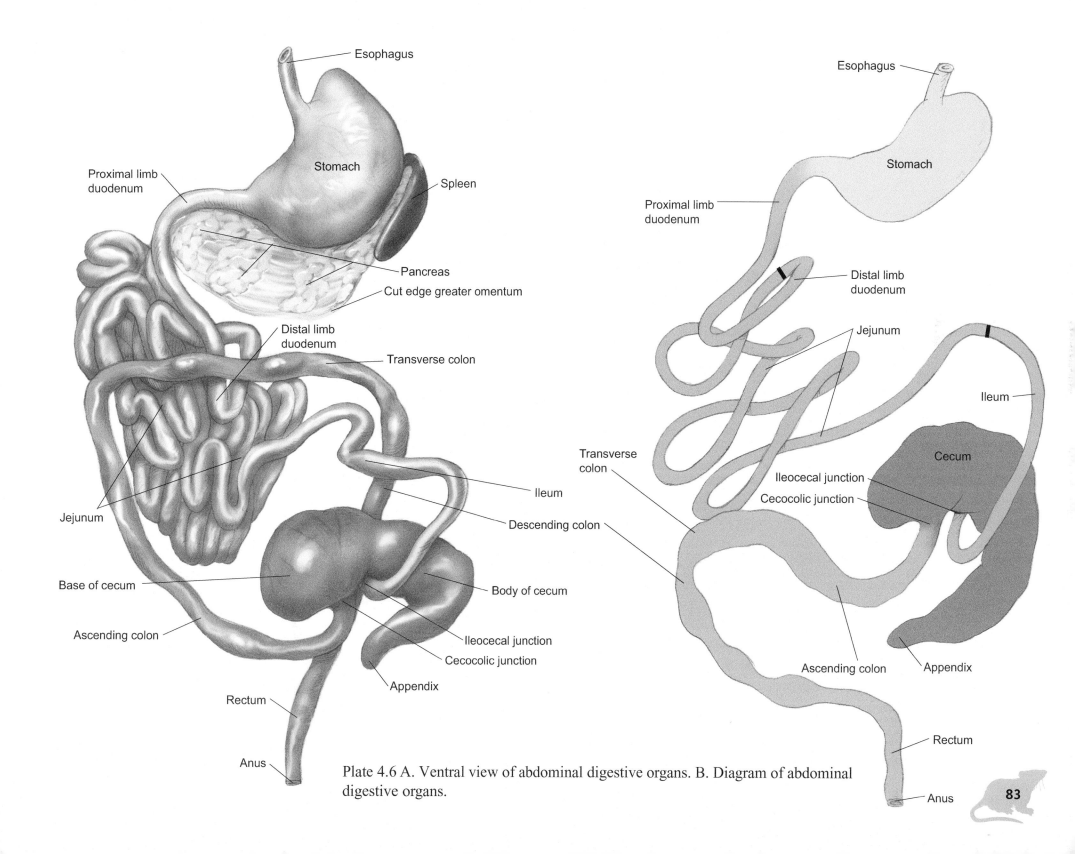

Esophagus

Proximal limb
duodenum

Stomach

Spleen

Pancreas

Cut edge greater omentum

Distal limb
duodenum

Transverse colon

Ileum

Descending colon

Jejunum

Body of cecum

Base of cecum

Ileocecal junction

Ascending colon

Cecocolic junction

Rectum

Appendix

Anus

Esophagus

Proximal limb
duodenum

Stomach

Distal limb
duodenum

Jejunum

Ileum

Transverse
colon

Cecum

Ileocecal junction

Cecocolic junction

Ascending colon

Appendix

Rectum

Anus

Plate 4.6 A. Ventral view of abdominal digestive organs. B. Diagram of abdominal
digestive organs.

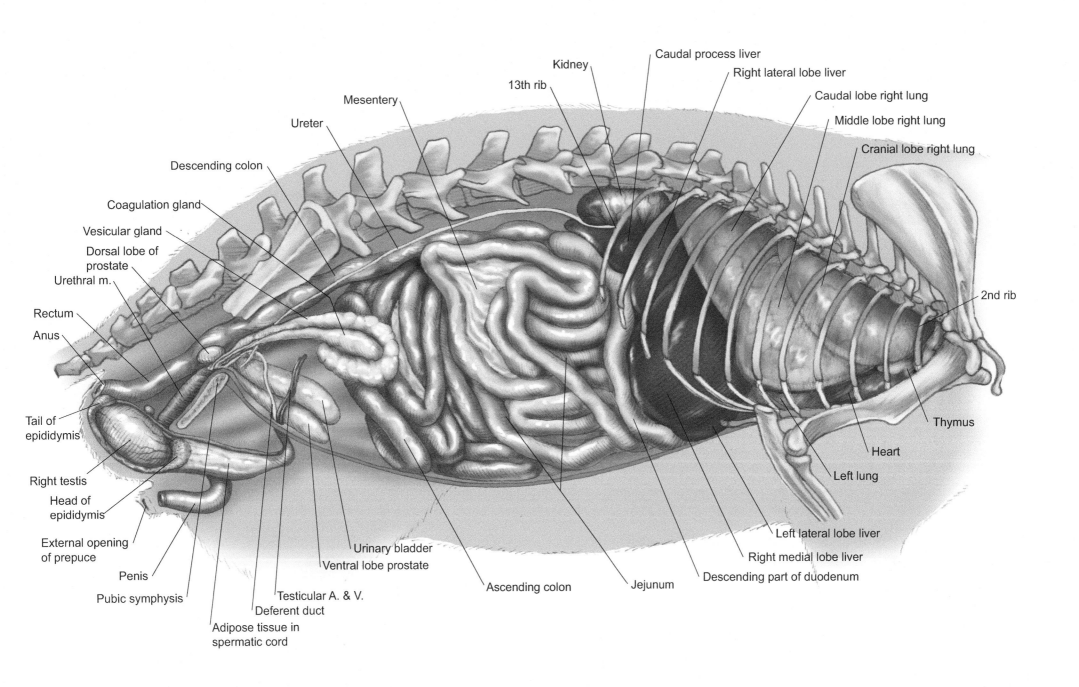

Plate 4.7 Right lateral view of thoracic, abdominal, and pelvic viscera of the male related to the skeleton.

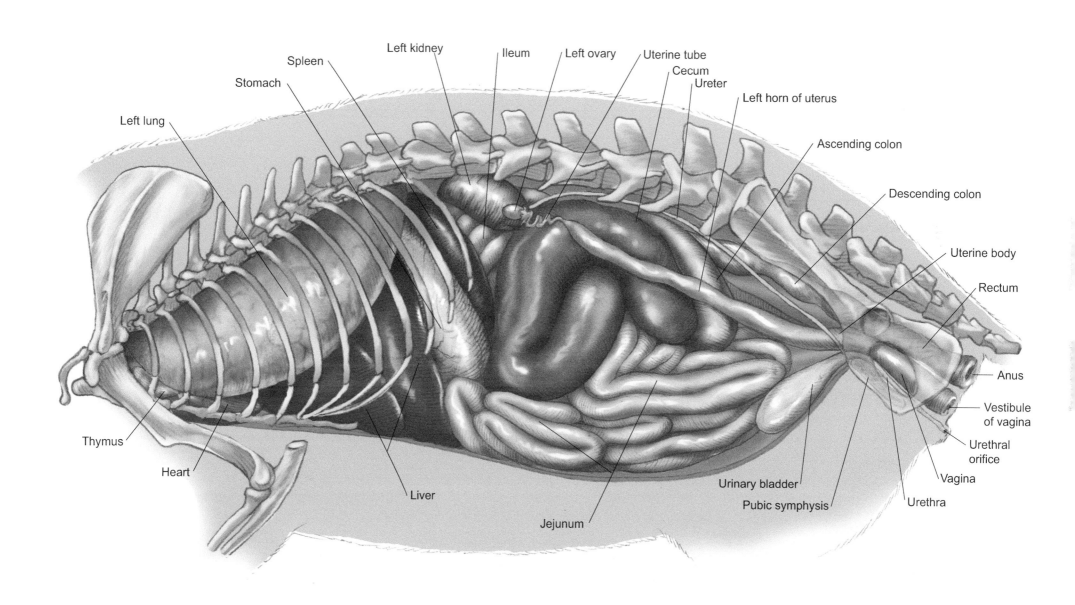

Plate 4.8 Left lateral view of thoracic, abdominal, and pelvic viscera of the female related to skeleton.

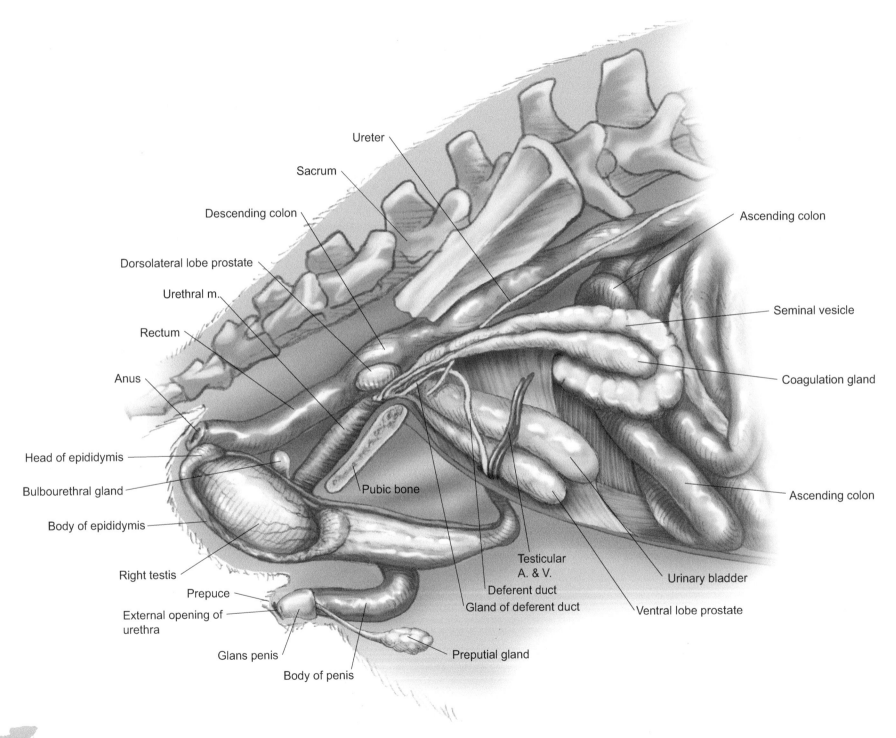

Ureter

Sacrum

Descending colon

Ascending colon

Dorsolateral lobe prostate

Urethral m.

Seminal vesicle

Rectum

Coagulation gland

Anus

Head of epididymis

Bulbourethral gland

Pubic bone

Ascending colon

Body of epididymis

Right testis

Testicular
A. & V.

Urinary bladder

Prepuce

Deferent duct

External opening of
urethra

Gland of deferent duct

Ventral lobe prostate

Glans penis

Body of penis

Preputial gland

Plate 4.9 Relations of the male reproductive organs.

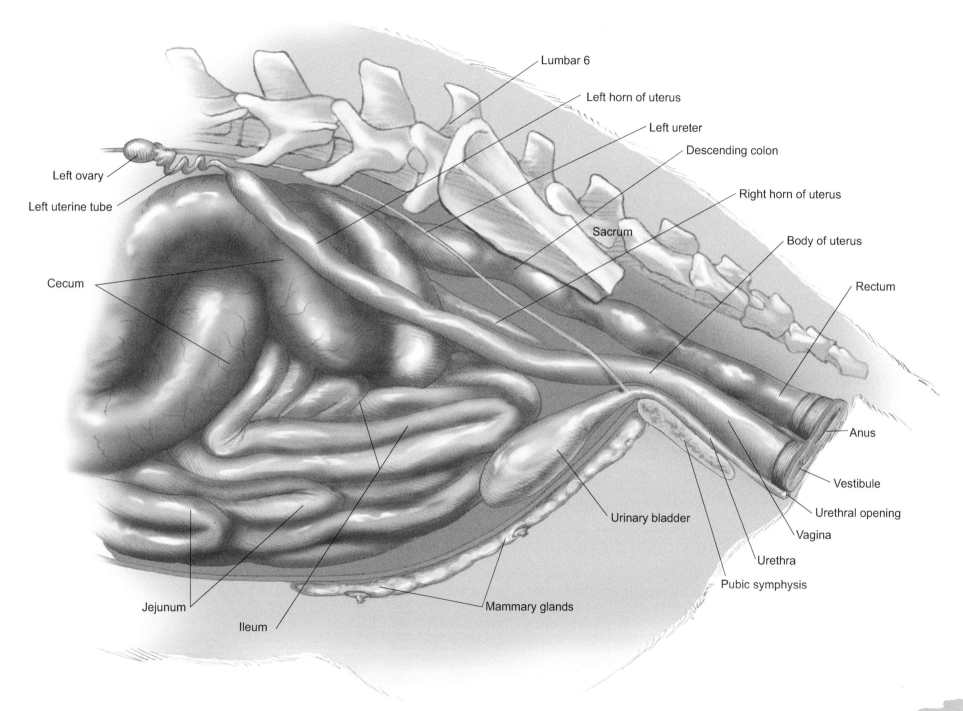

Lumbar 6

Left horn of uterus

Left ureter

Descending colon

Right horn of uterus

Body of uterus

Sacrum

Rectum

Left ovary

Left uterine tube

Cecum

Anus

Vestibule

Urethral opening

Urinary bladder

Vagina

Jejunum

Urethra

Ileum

Pubic symphysis

Mammary glands

Plate 4.10 Relations of the reproductive organs of the female.

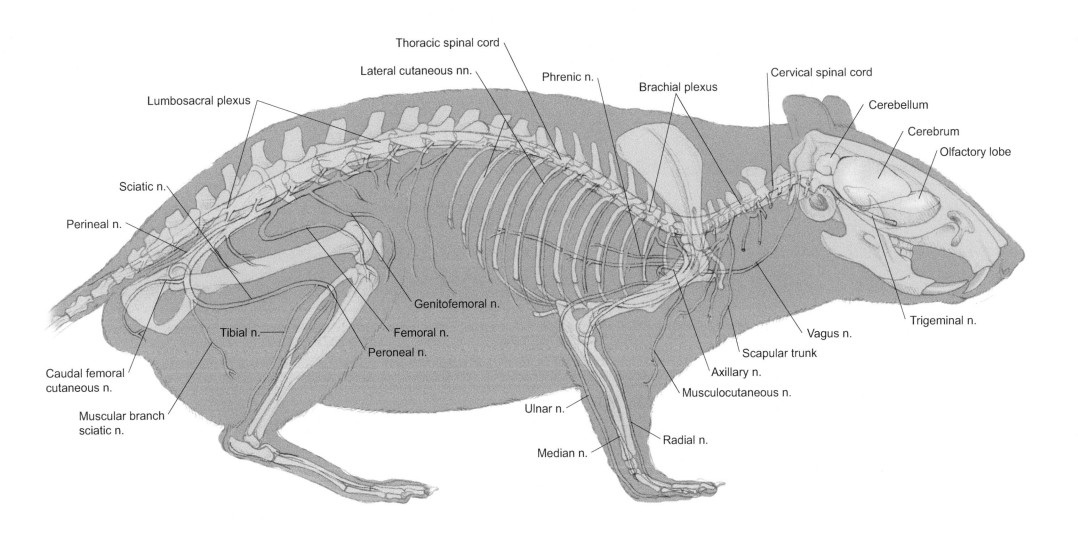

Plate 4.11 Central nervous system and peripheral nerves.

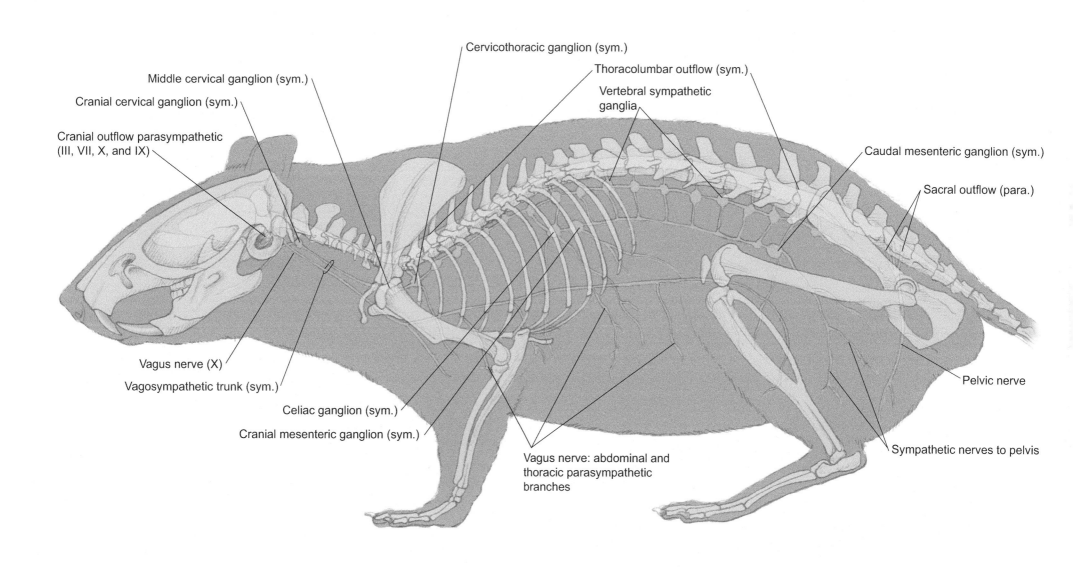

Cervicothoracic ganglion (sym.)

Thoracolumbar outflow (sym.)

Middle cervical ganglion (sym.)

Vertebral sympathetic ganglia

Cranial cervical ganglion (sym.)

Cranial outflow parasympathetic (III, VII, X, and IX)

Caudal mesenteric ganglion (sym.)

Sacral outflow (para.)

Vagus nerve (X)

Vagosympathetic trunk (sym.)

Celiac ganglion (sym.)

Cranial mesenteric ganglion (sym.)

Vagus nerve: abdominal and thoracic parasympathetic branches

Pelvic nerve

Sympathetic nerves to pelvis

Plate 4.12 Autonomic nerves: sym. = sympathetic division and para. = parasympathetic division.

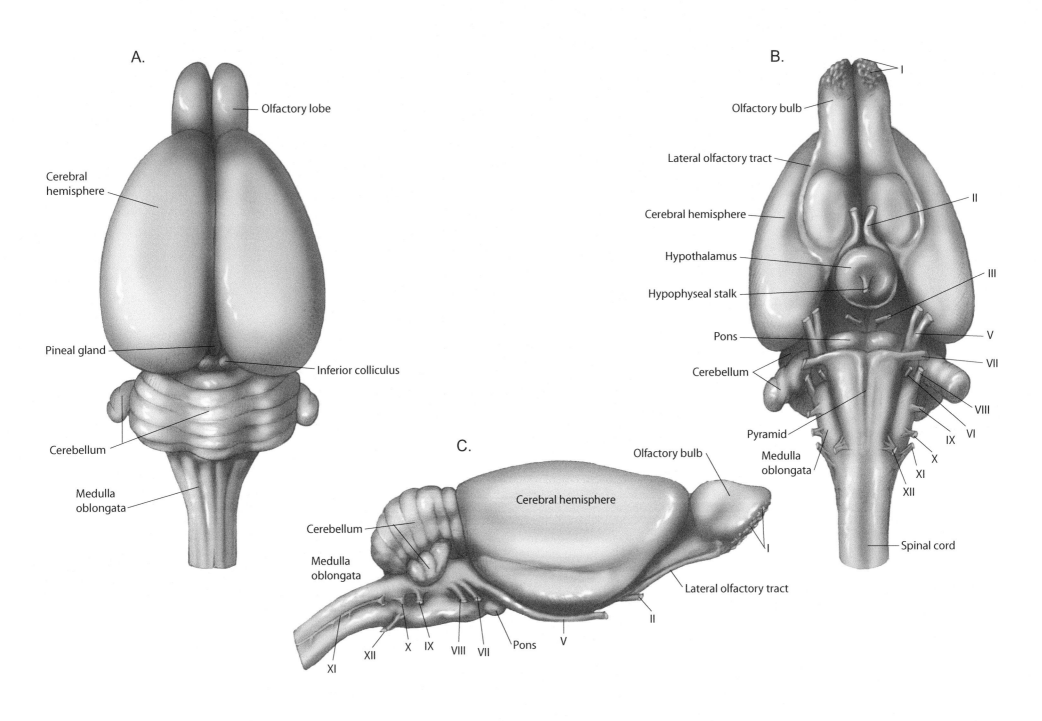

A.

Olfactory lobe

Cerebral hemisphere

Pineal gland

Inferior colliculus

Cerebellum

Medulla oblongata

B.

I

Olfactory bulb

Lateral olfactory tract

Cerebral hemisphere

Hypothalamus

Hypophyseal stalk

Pons

Cerebellum

Pyramid

Medulla oblongata

II

III

V

VII

VIII

VI

IX

X

XI

XII

Spinal cord

C.

Olfactory bulb

Cerebral hemisphere

Cerebellum

Medulla oblongata

I

Lateral olfactory tract

XI

XII

X

IX

VIII

VII

Pons

V

II

Plate 4.13 Brain: A. Dorsal view, B. Ventral view, C. Lateral view. I-olfactory, II-optic, III-oculomotor, V-trigeminal, VI-abducens, VII-facial, VIII-vestibulocochlear, IX-glossopharyngeal, X-vagus, XI-accessory, XII-hypoglossal nerves.

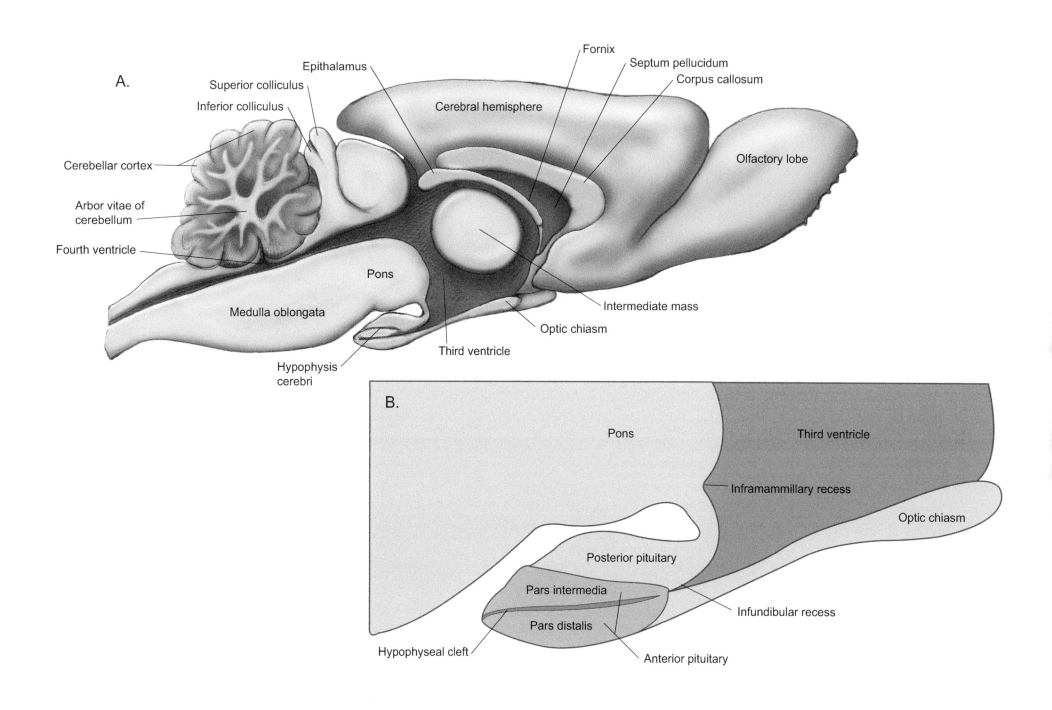

A.

Epithalamus

Superior colliculus

Inferior colliculus

Cerebellar cortex

Arbor vitae of cerebellum

Fourth ventricle

Medulla oblongata

Pons

Hypophysis cerebri

Third ventricle

Optic chiasm

Intermediate mass

Cerebral hemisphere

Fornix

Septum pellucidum

Corpus callosum

Olfactory lobe

B.

Pons

Third ventricle

Inframammillary recess

Optic chiasm

Posterior pituitary

Pars intermedia

Pars distalis

Infundibular recess

Hypophyseal cleft

Anterior pituitary

Plate 4.14 Brain: A. Midsagittal section, B. Detail of hypophysis.

SECTION 5 THE GUINEA PIG

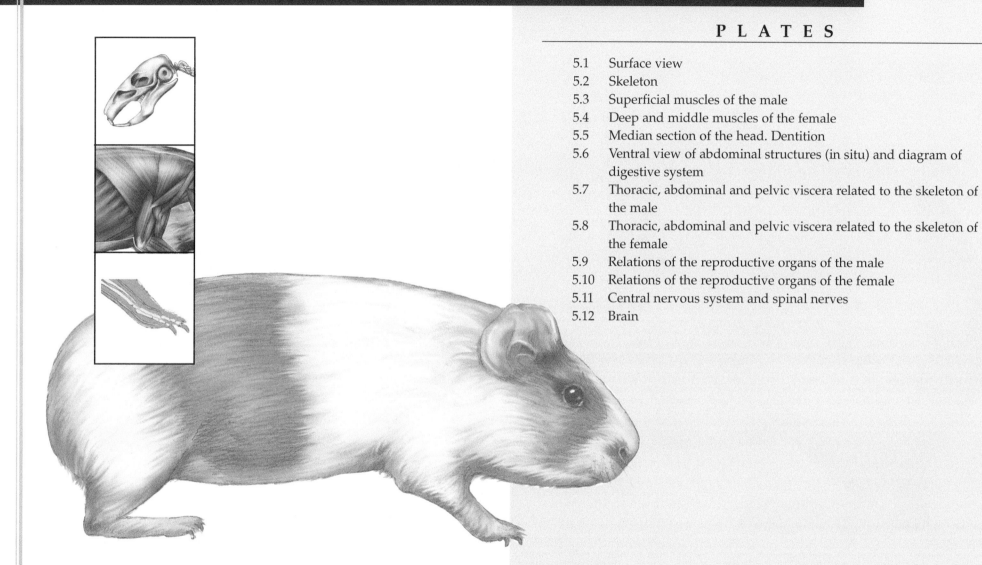

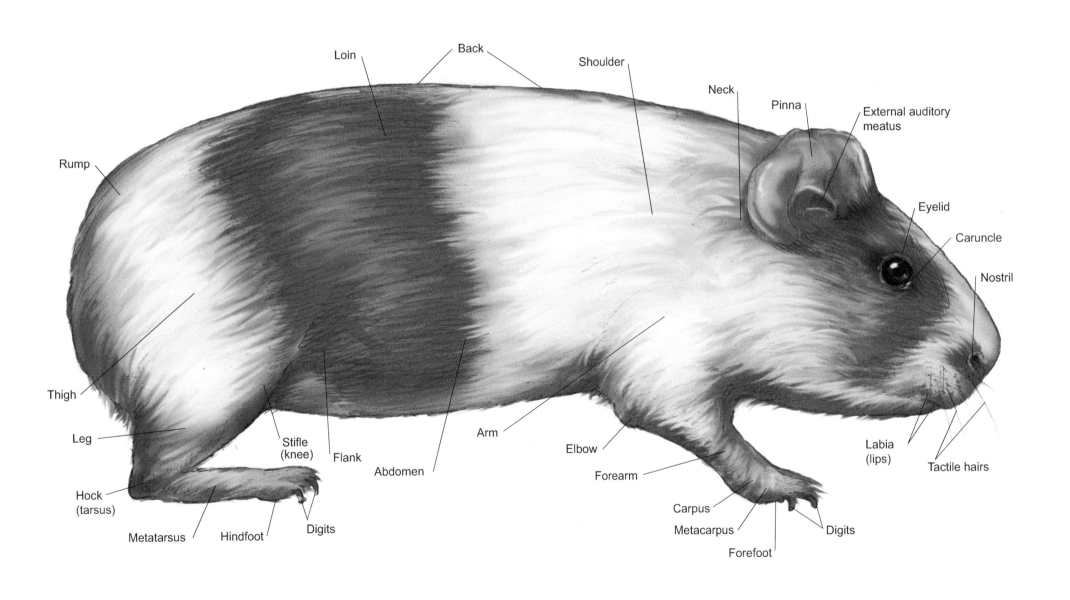

Loin

Back

Shoulder

Neck

Pinna

External auditory meatus

Rump

Eyelid

Caruncle

Nostril

Thigh

Arm

Leg

Elbow

Stifle (knee)

Labia (lips)

Flank

Forearm

Tactile hairs

Abdomen

Hock (tarsus)

Carpus

Metatarsus

Hindfoot

Digits

Metacarpus

Digits

Forefoot

Plate 5.1 Lateral view surface features.

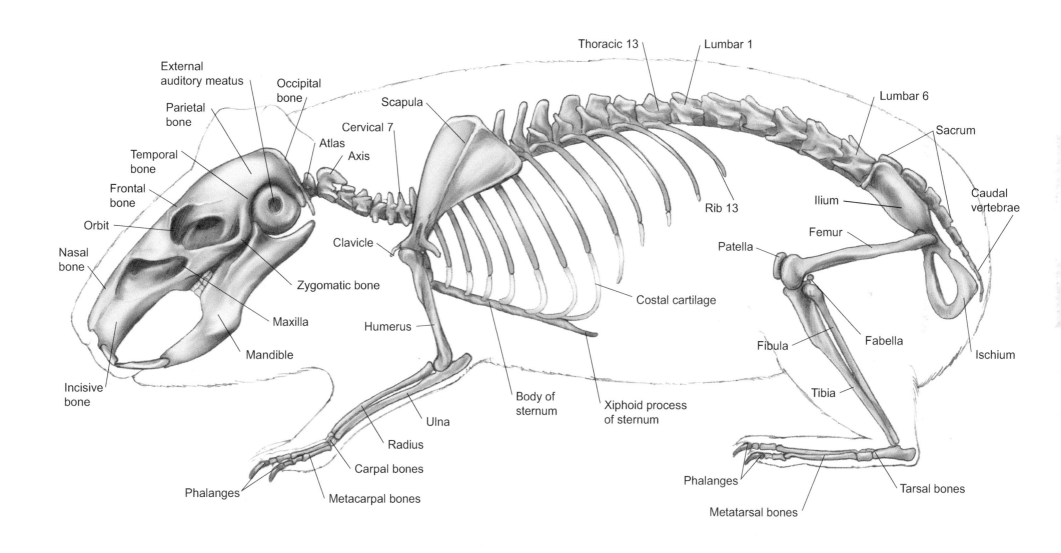

External
auditory meatus

Occipital
bone

Parietal
bone

Scapula

Thoracic 13

Lumbar 1

Lumbar 6

Temporal
bone

Cervical 7

Atlas

Axis

Sacrum

Frontal
bone

Orbit

Nasal
bone

Clavicle

Rib 13

Ilium

Caudal
vertebrae

Zygomatic bone

Patella

Femur

Incisive
bone

Maxilla

Mandible

Humerus

Costal cartilage

Fibula

Fabella

Ischium

Tibia

Body of
sternum

Xiphoid process
of sternum

Ulna

Radius

Carpal bones

Phalanges

Phalanges

Tarsal bones

Metacarpal bones

Metatarsal bones

Plate 5.2 Skeleton.

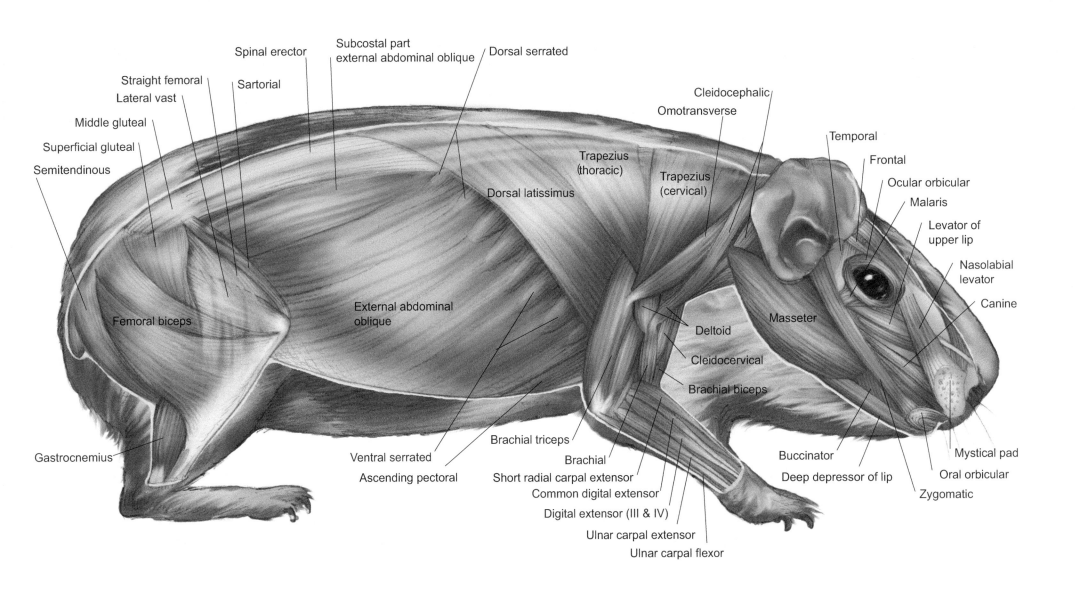

Plate 5.3 Lateral view of superficial muscles of the male.

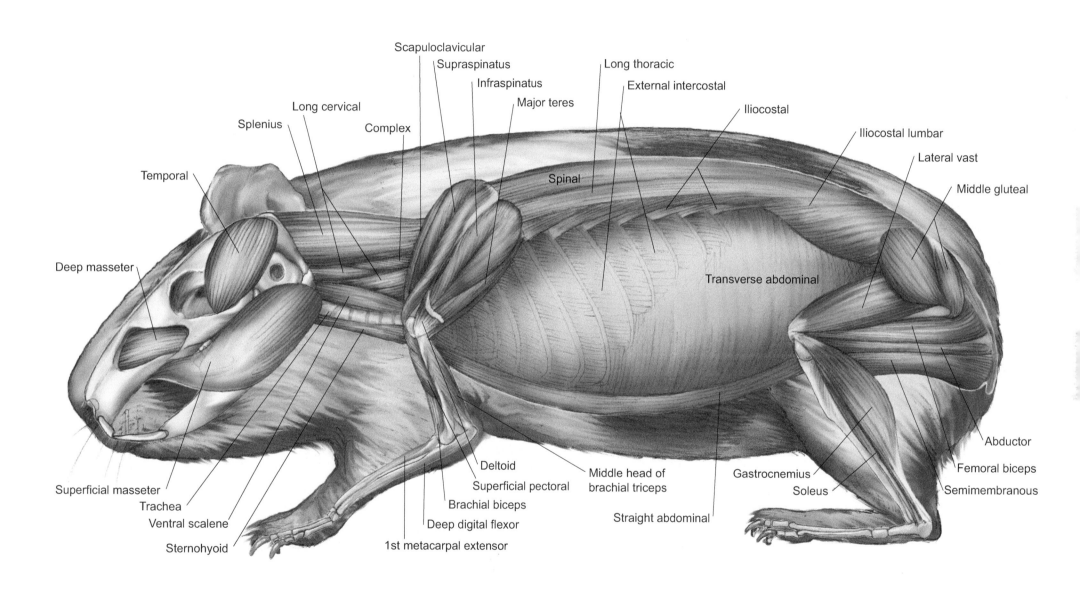

Scapuloclavicular
Supraspinatus
Infraspinatus
Major teres
Long thoracic
External intercostal
Iliocostal
Iliocostal lumbar
Lateral vast
Middle gluteal
Long cervical
Complex
Splenius
Spinal
Temporal
Deep masseter
Transverse abdominal
Superficial masseter
Trachea
Ventral scalene
Sternohyoid
Deltoid
Superficial pectoral
Brachial biceps
Deep digital flexor
1st metacarpal extensor
Middle head of
brachial triceps
Straight abdominal
Gastrocnemius
Soleus
Abductor
Femoral biceps
Semimembranous

Plate 5.4 Lateral view of deep muscles of the female.

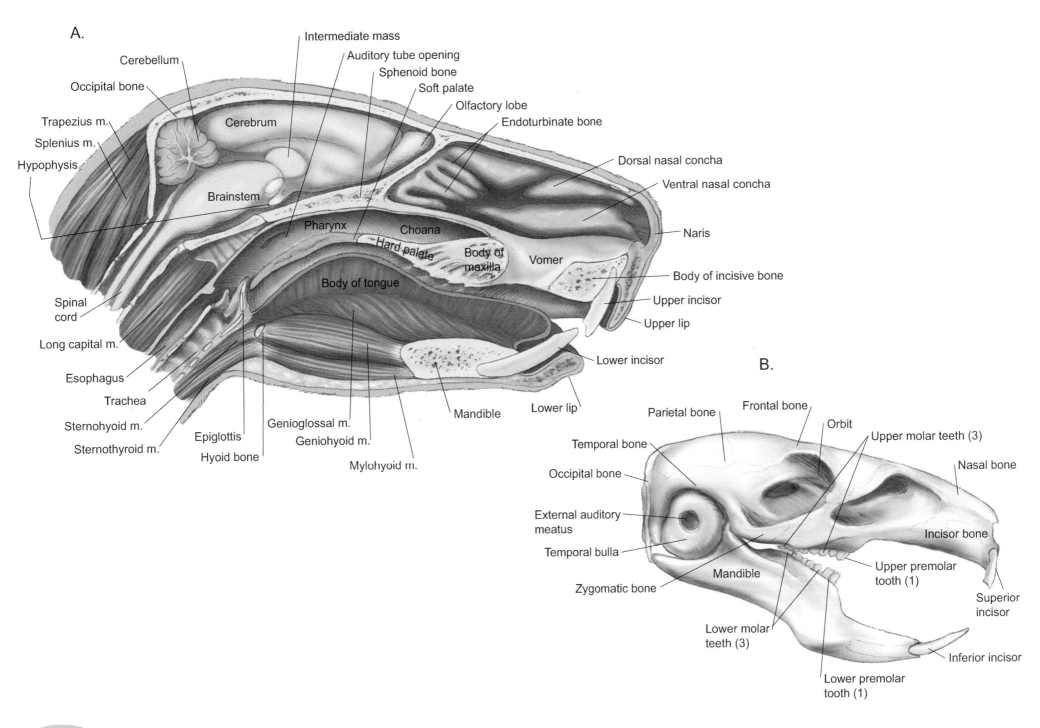

A.

Intermediate mass

Auditory tube opening

Cerebellum

Sphenoid bone

Occipital bone

Soft palate

Olfactory lobe

Trapezius m.

Cerebrum

Endoturbinate bone

Splenius m.

Dorsal nasal concha

Hypophysis

Ventral nasal concha

Brainstem

Spinal cord

Pharynx

Choana

Naris

Hard palate

Body of maxilla

Body of tongue

Vomer

Body of incisive bone

Upper incisor

Long capital m.

Upper lip

Esophagus

Lower incisor

Trachea

B.

Sternohyoid m.

Mandible

Lower lip

Sternothyroid m.

Epiglottis

Genioglossal m.

Hyoid bone

Geniohyoid m.

Mylohyoid m.

Parietal bone

Frontal bone

Orbit

Temporal bone

Upper molar teeth (3)

Occipital bone

Nasal bone

External auditory meatus

Incisor bone

Temporal bulla

Upper premolar tooth (1)

Zygomatic bone

Mandible

Superior incisor

Lower molar teeth (3)

Inferior incisor

Lower premolar tooth (1)

Plate 5.5 Head: A. Medial sagittal section, B. Skull and dentition.

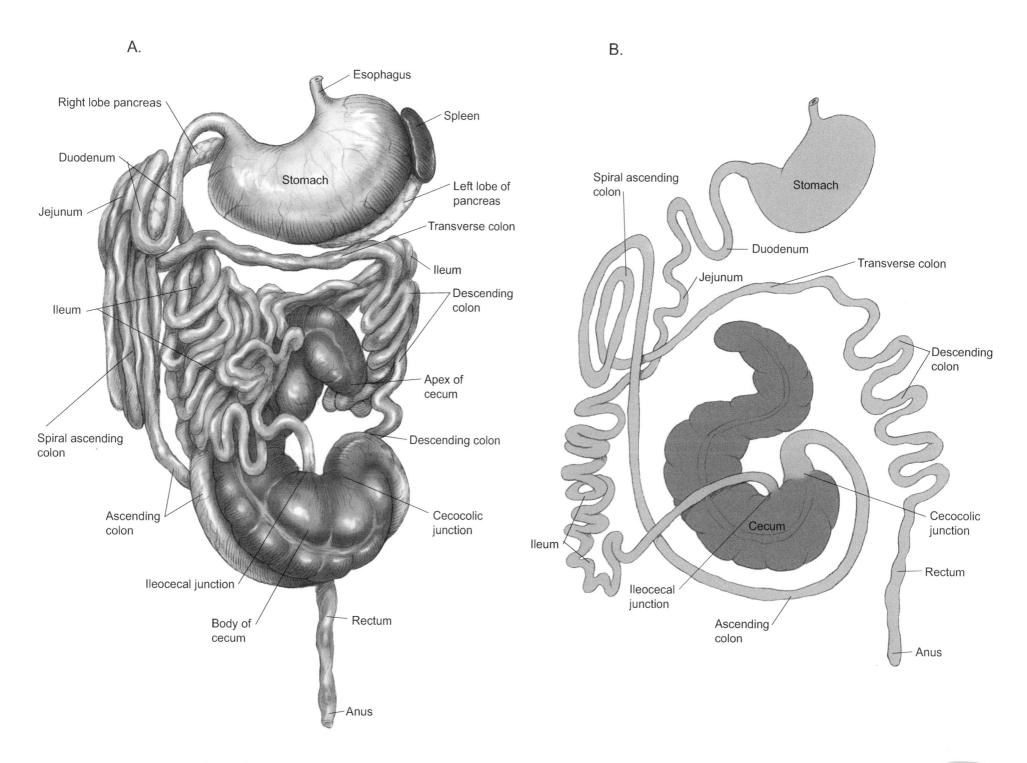

A.

Esophagus

Right lobe pancreas

Spleen

Duodenum

Stomach

Left lobe of pancreas

Jejunum

Transverse colon

Ileum

Ileum

Descending colon

Apex of cecum

Spiral ascending colon

Descending colon

Ascending colon

Cecocolic junction

Ileocecal junction

Body of cecum

Rectum

Anus

B.

Spiral ascending colon

Stomach

Duodenum

Jejunum

Transverse colon

Descending colon

Cecocolic junction

Ileum

Cecum

Rectum

Ileocecal junction

Ascending colon

Anus

Plate 5.6 Abdominal organs: A. Ventral view of abdominal organs (in situ), B. Diagram of digestive system.

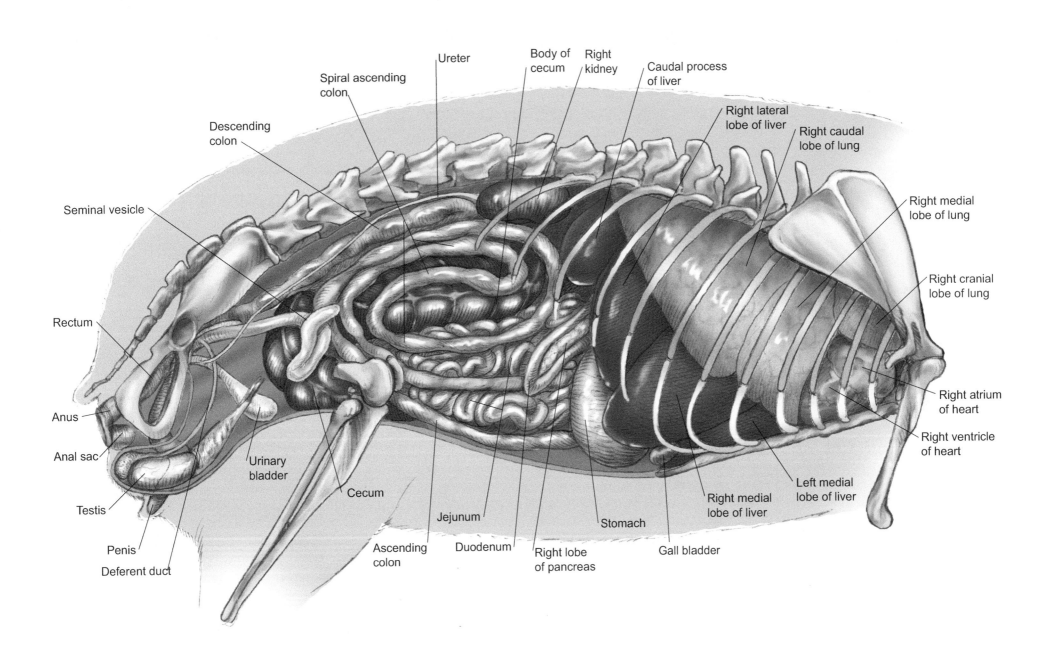

Ureter

Body of cecum

Right kidney

Caudal process of liver

Spiral ascending colon

Right lateral lobe of liver

Right caudal lobe of lung

Descending colon

Right medial lobe of lung

Seminal vesicle

Right cranial lobe of lung

Rectum

Right atrium of heart

Anus

Right ventricle of heart

Anal sac

Urinary bladder

Cecum

Testis

Left medial lobe of liver

Right medial lobe of liver

Jejunum

Stomach

Penis

Gall bladder

Deferent duct

Ascending colon

Duodenum

Right lobe of pancreas

Plate 5.7 Right lateral view of the thoracic, abdominal and pelvic viscera related to the skeleton of the male.

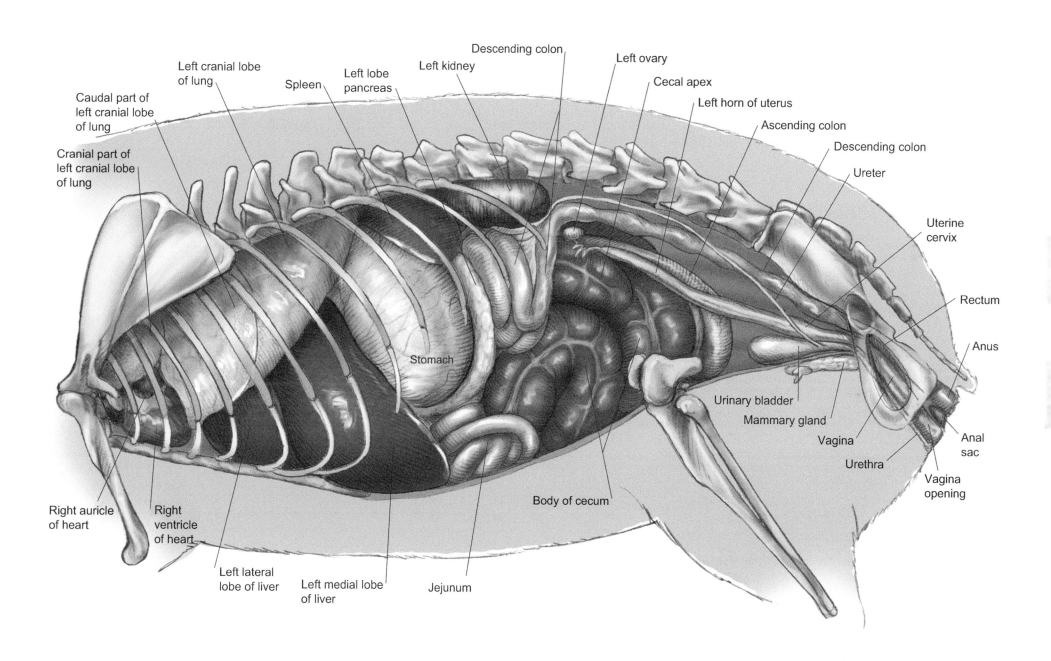

Plate 5.8 Left lateral view of the thoracic, abdominal and pelvic viscera related to the skeleton of the female.

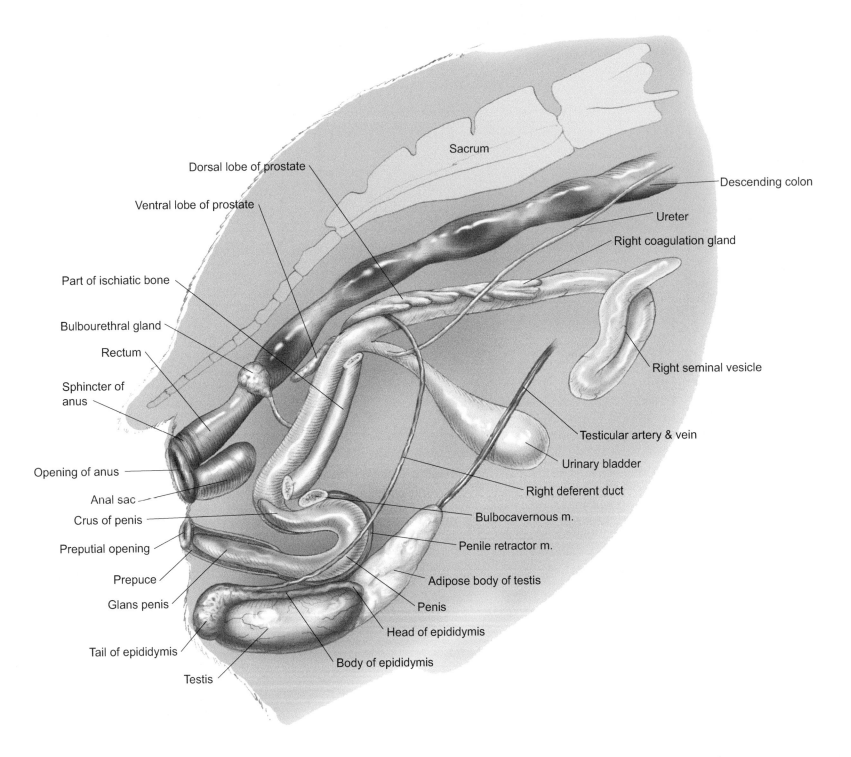

Dorsal lobe of prostate

Ventral lobe of prostate

Part of ischiatic bone

Bulbourethral gland

Rectum

Sphincter of anus

Opening of anus

Anal sac

Crus of penis

Preputial opening

Prepuce

Glans penis

Tail of epididymis

Testis

Sacrum

Descending colon

Ureter

Right coagulation gland

Right seminal vesicle

Testicular artery & vein

Urinary bladder

Right deferent duct

Bulbocavernous m.

Penile retractor m.

Adipose body of testis

Penis

Head of epididymis

Body of epididymis

Plate 5.9 Relations of the reproductive organs of the male.

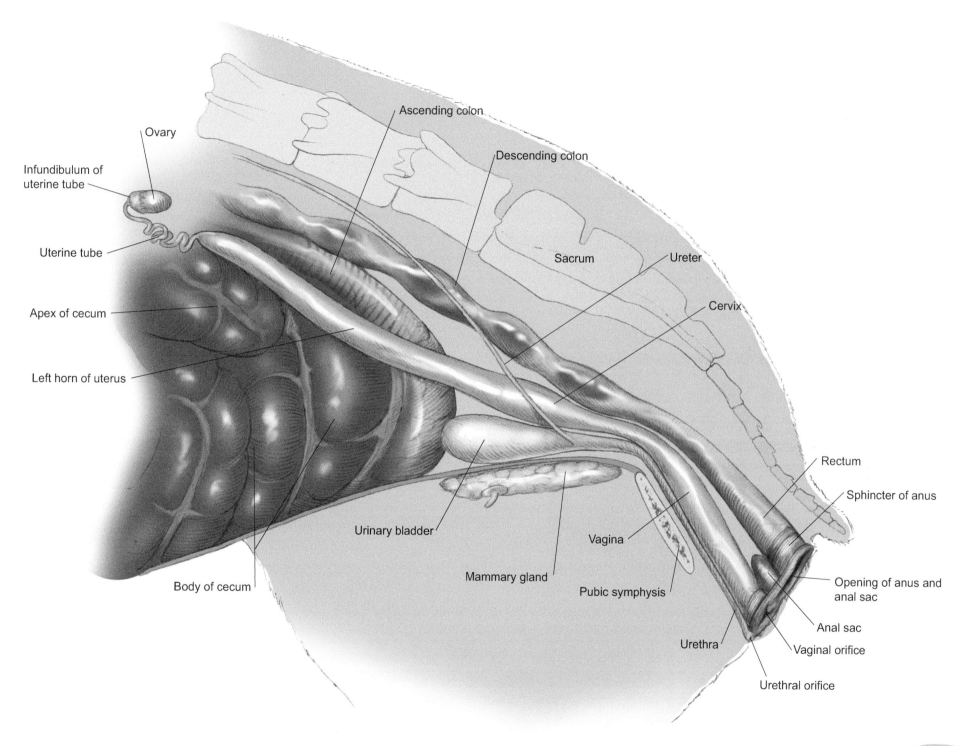

Plate 5.10 Left lateral view of the relations of the reproductive organs of the female.

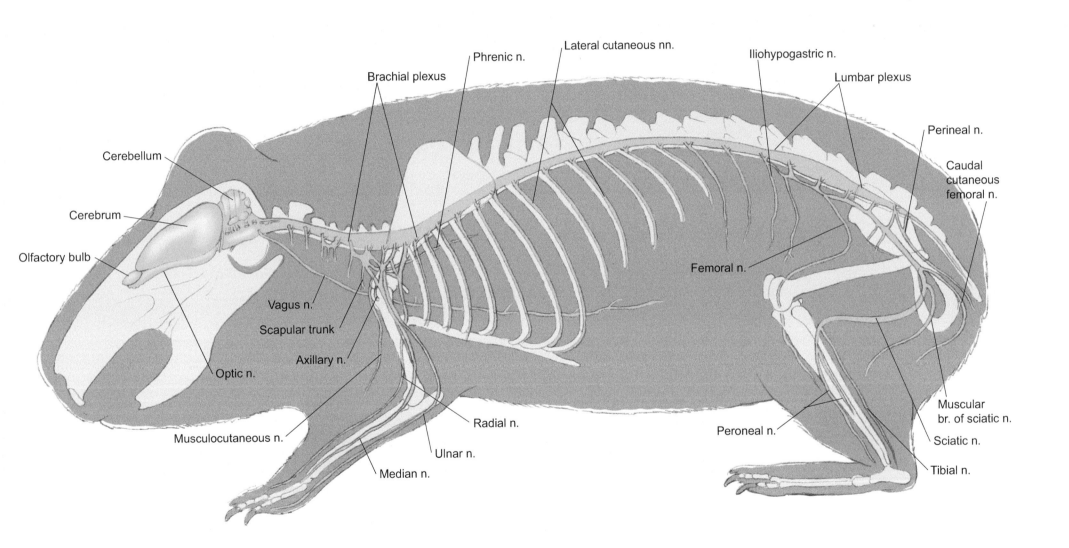

Cerebellum

Cerebrum

Olfactory bulb

Optic n.

Brachial plexus

Phrenic n.

Lateral cutaneous nn.

Iliohypogastric n.

Lumbar plexus

Perineal n.

Caudal cutaneous femoral n.

Femoral n.

Vagus n.

Scapular trunk

Axillary n.

Musculocutaneous n.

Radial n.

Ulnar n.

Median n.

Peroneal n.

Muscular br. of sciatic n.

Sciatic n.

Tibial n.

104

Plate 5.11 Central and peripheral nervous systems.

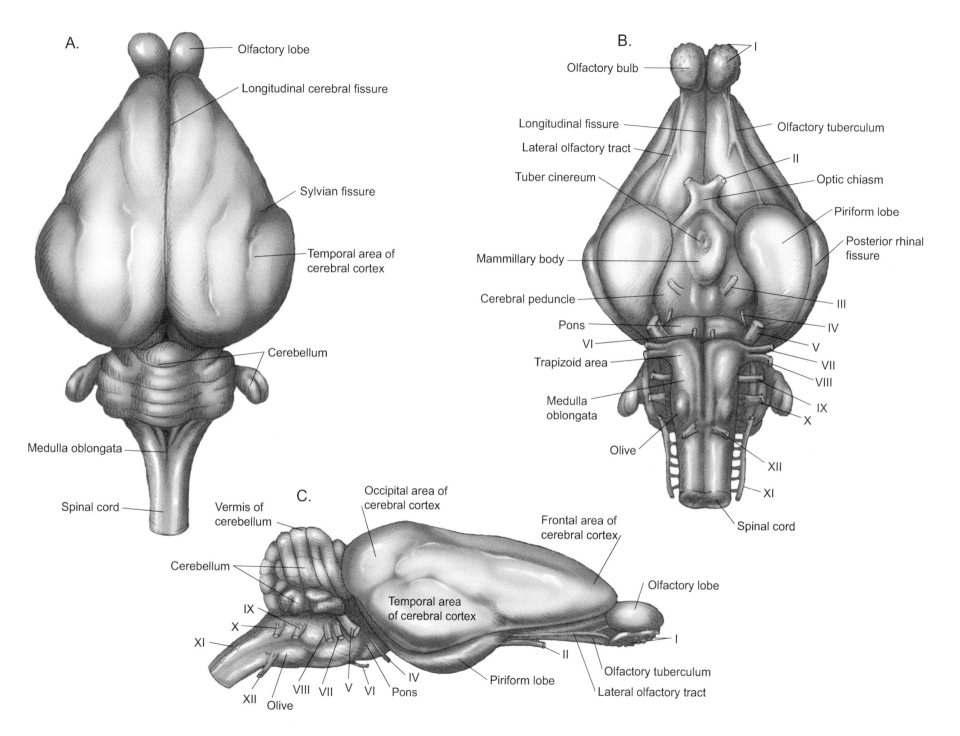

A. Dorsal view

- Olfactory lobe
- Longitudinal cerebral fissure
- Sylvian fissure
- Temporal area of cerebral cortex
- Cerebellum
- Medulla oblongata
- Spinal cord

B. Ventral view

- I
- Olfactory bulb
- Longitudinal fissure
- Olfactory tuberculum
- Lateral olfactory tract
- II
- Tuber cinereum
- Optic chiasm
- Piriform lobe
- Mammillary body
- Posterior rhinal fissure
- Cerebral peduncle
- III
- Pons
- IV
- VI
- V
- Trapizoid area
- VII
- VIII
- Medulla oblongata
- IX
- X
- Olive
- XII
- XI
- Spinal cord

C. Lateral view

- Occipital area of cerebral cortex
- Vermis of cerebellum
- Frontal area of cerebral cortex
- Cerebellum
- Olfactory lobe
- IX
- Temporal area of cerebral cortex
- X
- XI
- II
- Olfactory tuberculum
- Lateral olfactory tract
- XII
- Olive
- VIII
- VII
- V
- VI
- Pons
- IV
- Piriform lobe

Plate 5.12 Brain: A. Dorsal view, B. Ventral view, C. Lateral view. I-olfactory, II-optic, III-oculomotor, IV-trochlear, V-trigeminal, VI-abducens, VII-facial, VIII-vestibulocochlear, IX-glossopharyngeal, X-vagus, XI-hypoglossal, XII-accessory nerves.

INDEX

Buccinator
   dog, 7
   guinea pig, 96
   rabbit, 66
   rat, 80
Bulbocavernous muscle, guinea pig, 102
Bulbospongious muscle
   cat, 52
   dog, 18, 24
Bulbourethral gland
   cat, 50, 52
   guinea pig, 102
   rabbit, 70, 72
   rat, 86

C

Canine muscle
   guinea pig, 96
   rabbit, 66
   rat, 80
Canine teeth
   cat, 42
   dog, 12
Capital muscles
   cranial oblique, cat, 42
   long
      cat, 42
      dog, 9, 12
      guinea pig, 98
      rabbit, 68
      rat, 81
   longest
      dog, 9
      rabbit, 68
   rhomboid
      dog, 8
      rat, 80, 81
Capsular muscle, cat, 41
Carotid artery
   cat, 55
   dog, 27
Carpal bones
   cat, 37

dog, 5
   guinea pig, 95
   rabbit, 64
   rat, 79
Carpal extensors
   dog, 8
   rabbit, 67
Carpal flexors, rabbit, 67
Carpal pads
   cat, 48, 49
   dog, 11
Carpal region
   cat, 36
   dog, 4
   rabbit, 63
Carpus
   cat, 34
   dog, 2, 3
   guinea pig, 94
   rabbit, 62
Caruncle, guinea pig, 94
Cat, xiii-xiv
   abdomen, 34, 50, 51
   arteries, 55
   autonomic nervous system, 58
   body regions, 36
   brain, 42, 59
   central nervous system, 42, 57, 59
   cervical nerves, 59
   dentition, 42
   digits, 48, 49
   ear, 44
   endocrine organs, 56
   eye, 45
   fasciae, 38
   female
      genitourinary system, 41, 51, 53
      lateral view, 35, 50
      viscera, 41
   forepaw, 48, 49
   gastrointestinal system, 46, 47, 50, 51
   head, 40, 42
   hindpaw, 49
   kidney, 41, 50

J

M

N

Optic chiasm
cat, 59
dog, 31
guinea pig, 105
rat, 82, 91
Optic nerve
cat, 45
dog, 31
guinea pig, 104
Optic retina, cat, 45
Oral cavity
cat, 43
rabbit, 68
Oral orbicular muscle
cat, 39
dog, 7
guinea pig, 96
rabbit, 66
rat, 81
Orbit
dog, 2
guinea pig, 95, 98
rabbit, 62
Oropharynx, dog, 12
Os coxae, guinea pig, 95
Ovarian artery/vein, cat, 55
Ovarian duct, cat, 41
Ovary
cat, 41, 51, 56
dog, 9, 21, 23
guinea pig, 101, 103
rabbit, 65, 71, 73
rat, 85, 87

P

Palatine process
dog, 14
rabbit, 68
Palatopharyngeal arch, cat, 43
Palmar, xvi, xvii, 35
Palmar anular ligament, dog, 10
Palpebral artery, cat, 55
Palpebral depressor, rabbit, 66

Pancreas
cat, 56
dog, 19, 20, 23
guinea pig, 99, 100, 101
rabbit, 65, 70
rat, 83
Pancreatic duct, cat, 46
Pancreatic lymph nodes, rabbit, 65
Papillae
duodenal, cat, 46, 47
tongue
cat, 43
dog, 16
rabbit, 69
Parasympathetic nerves
cat, 58
dog, 30
rat, 89
Parathyroid gland
cat, 56
dog, 23
Parietal bone
cat, 37, 42
dog, 5, 12
guinea pig, 95, 98
rabbit, 64, 68
rat, 79
Parietal pericardium, xx, xxi
dog, 19
Parietal peritoneum, xx, xxi
dog, 19
Parietal pleura, xx, xxi
dog, 19
Parotid gland, dog, 15
Parotid lymph nodes
cat, 56
dog, 28
rabbit, 65
Parotidoauricular muscle, dog, 7
Parotidomandibular muscle, cat, 39
Pars distalis, rat, 91
Pars intermedia, rat, 91
Pastern, cat, 34

Reproductive organs (*continued*)

    guinea pig

        female, 103

        male, 102

    rabbit

        female, 73

        male, 72

    rat

        female, 85, 87

        male, 84, 86

Rete mirabile, cat, 55

Retina

    cat eye, 45

    dog eye, 13

Retractor penis

    cat, 52

    dog, 18

    rabbit, 72

Retropharyngeal lymph nodes

    cat, 56

    dog, 28

Rhomboid muscles

    capital

        dog, 8

        rat, 80, 81

    cervical

        cat, 40

        dog, 8

        rabbit, 67

        rat, 81

Ribs

    cat, 37

    dog, 5

    guinea pig, 95

    rabbit, 64

    rat, 79, 84

Roof rat, xiv

Rostral, xvi, xvii, 35

Rump

    guinea pig, 94

    rabbit, 62

    rat, 78

S

Sacral arteries, cat, 55

Sacral lymph nodes, cat, 56

Sacral outflow

    cat, 58

    dog, 30

    rat, 89

Sacral region

    cat, 36

    dog, 4

    rabbit, 63

Sacral tuber, dog, 22

Sacral veins, cat, 54

Sacral vertebrae

    cat, 37

    rat, 79

Sacrocaudal muscles

    cat, 39

    dog, 7, 8

Sacroiliac joints, dog, 22

Sacroiliac ligament, dog, 22

Sacrotuberous ligament, dog, 22

Sacrum

    dog, 22

    guinea pig, 95

    rabbit, 64

    rat, 86, 87

Sagittal plane, xviii, xix

Saphenous artery

    cat, 55

    dog, 27

Saphenous nerve, dog, 29

Saphenous vein

    cat, 54

    dog, 26

Sartorius muscle

    cat, 39

    dog, 7, 8

    guinea pig, 96

Scalene muscles

    guinea pig, 97

    rat, 81

Scapula

    cat, 37

136